Extraordinary Healers

CURE Readers Honor Oncology Nurses

Volume 7

Extraordinary Healers

CURE Readers Honor Oncology Nurses

Volume 7

curemedia**group**

Dallas, Texas

Made possible with financial support from

Amgen, Inc.

Millennium: The Takeda Oncology Company.

Published by
CURE Media Group
3102 Oak Lawn, Suite 610
Dallas, Texas 75219
curemagazine.com

Information presented is not intended as a substitute for the personalized professional advice given by a healthcare provider. This publication was produced by CURE Media Group. The views expressed in this publication are not necessarily those of the publisher. Although great care has been taken to ensure accuracy, CURE Media Group and its servants or agents shall not be responsible or in any way liable for the continued currency of the information or for any errors, omissions or inaccuracies in this book, whether arising from negligence or otherwise, or for any consequences arising therefrom. The intention of this book is not to provide specific medical advice; therefore, all references to specific commercial products have been removed. Essays have also been edited for grammar, style, length and clarity. Review and creation of content is solely the responsibility of CURE Media Group.

Any mention of retail products does not constitute an endorsement by the authors or the publisher.

Library of Congress Control Number: 2014931162

ISBN 9780985911447

Edited by Katherine Lagomarsino
Designed by Susan Douglass
Layout by Glenn Zamora
Photo Coordination by Erin Moore and Glenn Zamora
Event Coordination by Alexandra Hurd

Printed in the United States of America

This book is dedicated to all oncology nurses who bring hope and healing to cancer patients and their loved ones.

If you would like to give this book as a gift to your Extraordinary Healer, we've provided this page for your message.

This book honors:

_____

_____

_____

_____

_____

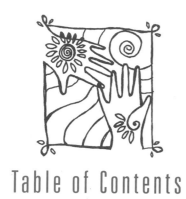

Table of Contents

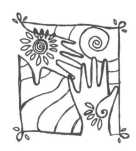

Why Oncology Nursing?

JUST AS I AM SURPRISED WHY ANY DOCTOR would want to be an oncologist, I have been equally surprised why nurses would want to work in oncology.

Until I figured it out.

Let's face it, oncology is hard. Patients are diagnosed with the scourge of the 21st century. And we often aren't very nice, having been shocked into mortality by the word "cancer." Why would anyone want to specialize in an area of medicine where the patients are sick and, for the most part, have to go through difficult treatment to get better?

As a longtime survivor, having been diagnosed with breast cancer in 1986 at age 37, I have listened to and observed oncology nurses for many years. It's like I could write the oncology nurse job description, which would ask for someone with strong medical credentials with the patience of a saint and a depth of feeling few have. Every year when the *Extraordinary Healer* essays start coming in from around the country, I begin reading them with knowledge of what they will say and the people they will honor.

Over the years I have also had the chance to speak at Oncology Nursing Society meetings around the country. I may address issues such as medical adherence or perform my one-woman show about cancer. The show is designed for laughter, with some subtle descriptions about the bizarre things we patients share. Oncology nurses are the hardest audience. I have to work to get them into the present to enjoy their time and not dwell on the lives of their patients in the past.

I start my presentation by passing out tablets and asking the nurses to describe why they chose oncology nursing. There is no hesitation with this task; they begin writing in earnest.

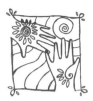

They know why they became oncology nurses—and most can recount the exact moment they knew. After I ask them to stop writing, I say casually that I know what they have written on the paper.

"You became oncology nurses for the money, right?" I say to a chorus of chortles. "Oh, that's right," I correct myself. "It's the hours. You like those hours." Now they are really looking at me as if I'm crazy, except for the few who are catching on. The next one always gets to them.

"No?" I ask. "Then it must be your affinity for body fluids."

Now they laugh and poke each other. "Sure," says one longtime oncology nurse. "I love vomit."

Then I love to surprise them, because next I say that I really do know what they have written. They all look around and turn their sheet over as if I have been reading over their shoulder. So I continue.

With few exceptions, I tell them, there are two reasons they became oncology nurses. First, they had lived through a cancer diagnosis with someone they cared about and were compelled to become oncology nurses to alleviate the suffering they knew so well. Many of them carry that person with them, and there are tears as they remember the mother, father, sister, brother, best friend or neighbor.

Or, I continue, you vowed after nursing school and a round in oncology, you would never work in oncology. You hated it. Then there was a circumstance that required that you work in oncology. Like the nurse who took a maternity leave only to learn on returning to work that there were no openings except in oncology.

Or the nurse who relocated with her husband to a new city and discovered that the closest hospital was a cancer center, so a job there would allow her extra hours in the day because she wouldn't have to commute.

It was hopeless, I tell them, because I am sure they know by now that they had been chosen early in life to care for those with cancer. It is not a job, it is a calling. And they have been called.

—Kathy LaTour, *CURE*'s Editor-at-Large

Extraordinary Healers
Our Winner
& Finalists

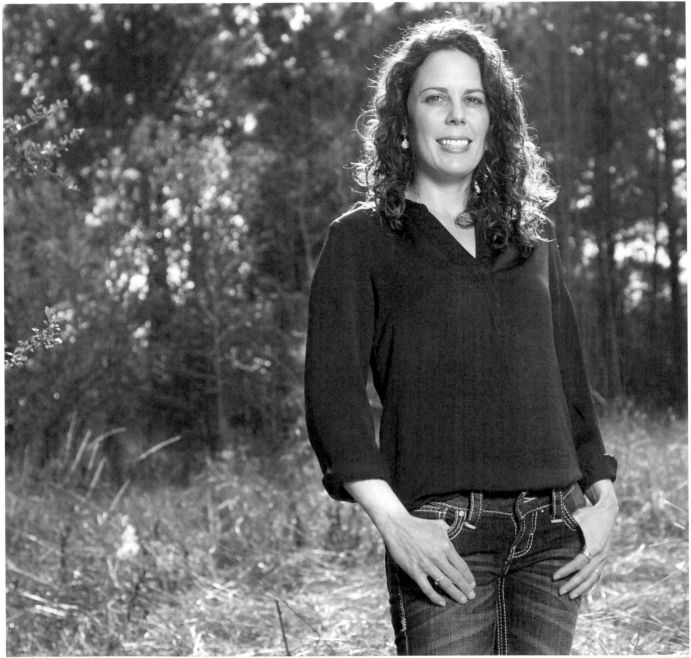

Angela Krach, RN, BSN

Transcending Cure With Care

WINNER OF THE 2013 EXTRAORDINARY HEALER AWARD FOR ONCOLOGY NURSING

ANGELA KRACH, RN, BSN [MD ANDERSON CANCER CENTER IN HOUSTON]

WRITTEN BY ANNE FALGOUST OTT

IT IS DIFFICULT to stand out, head and shoulders above the other nurses at an institution of MD Anderson's magnitude, but Angela Krach does stand out—not only for her exceptional clinical skills but also for her compassion and commitment to my husband and me.

ON MARCH 30, 2012, my then-fiancé James called midafternoon, slightly panicked, saying his doctor had just told him to go directly to an emergency room—all his blood cell counts were dangerously low, and it could not wait through the weekend. James had not been feeling well overall and got unusually winded on a walk the day before, prompting him to go see his doctor. We had no idea what that meant at the time, but six hours later, doctors hospitalized James and told us he likely had leukemia. We were in complete and utter shock, and our lives took a 180-degree turn. Just the night before I had been bugging James to decide if he wanted to wear tails or a tuxedo to our wedding that was planned for a few months later, in August 2012; now we were planning to battle for his life.

James' leukemia was one of the more dire subsets that required a bone marrow transplantation for a chance to live; however, his insurance company would only cover the requisite stem cell transplantation at a "center of excellence." So we transferred our lives to Houston and MD Anderson and ended up under the attentive care of Angela Krach. We met Angela when James was readmitted to the hospital in November 2012 for complications following his August stem cell transplantation.

Expected complications, such as graft-versus-host disease, and some not-so-expected complications, such as viral encephalitis and a suspected fungal pneumonia, created a perfect storm for James, who has been in the hospital for the past four and a half months, with the exception of 14 days just before Christmas. Angela admitted James that first night, when he transferred from the Ambulatory Treatment Center to the inpatient stem cell transplantation unit. She was welcoming and clinically efficient in those first 24 hours, but it was not until later that we discovered her truly exceptional professional and personal intuition.

As James' encephalitis started to resolve and he resumed eating again, he began experiencing a delayed cough. Angela was the first to note that the cough might be more than it seemed, suspecting that he was silently aspirating. She persistently approached the medical team to advocate for a chest X-ray and barium swallow test, which not only confirmed that he was silently aspirating but also that he had developed aspiration pneumonitis. Her insistence led to interventions for James that kept him alive and in a rehabilitative state. It is her ability to go beyond the everyday responsibilities of nursing and to use a professional's intuition to anticipate problems that make her such an exceptional clinician.

That was not an isolated occurrence. A few weeks later, James was extremely lethargic and fatigued, and Angela quickly assessed that his oxygen saturation was dangerously abnormal. She immediately intervened and, within moments, had an entire team of professionals at his bedside to transition James to the intensive care unit where his pulmonary function could be better monitored. He was later diagnosed with pneumonia that the doctors suspected was fungal.

TEACHING MOMENT:

She orchestrated a dress rehearsal for James two days before the wedding, carefully camouflaging his catheter and other tubing on the wheelchair and ensuring that he was fully dressed in his tuxedo.

Angela also went above and beyond to make sure James was progressing physically. She was right there for him, with a smile underneath her mask, an unmatched energy and a can-do attitude. She didn't simply administer medications; she was willing to attend to his global care needs, including physical therapy work. Sadly, James was bedridden and had to be prompted to do the various exercises he had to do each day to get better. Angela was the only nurse who consistently found a way to engage him in a way he responded to: the results were tangible when she cared for him. I credit her with kick-starting James' recovery, pushing him to do more each day and recognizing when she should nudge him a bit more. She also took time to make sure I understood everything that went on with James medically. She eased my fears and even checked on us after her shifts, when she wasn't our nurse, to see how we were doing.

Though many nominations likely include stories of nurses who go above and beyond to clinically support their patients, what sets Angela apart even further was her help in making our wedding day perfect and special—even in the hospital. James and I originally planned our wedding for August 2012; after he was diagnosed, we decided we would get married when we returned home after his transplantation. We have yet to return home, and it is still unclear when he might leave the hospital. But we had been through so much together this past year and no longer wanted to wait to say, "I do." We arranged to have our wedding and reception at MD Anderson, and Angela was instrumental in making our dream a reality. She orchestrated a dress rehearsal for James two days before the wedding, carefully camouflaging his catheter and other tubing on the wheelchair and ensuring that he was fully dressed in his tuxedo. She was off the day of our wedding but came to the hospital to dress him and made him feel and appear the perfect groom. She gave him some of his dignity back by ensuring he looked his best in front of family and friends and celebrated with us as a member of our now-extended MD Anderson family. It is impossible to convey the magnitude of what her kindness meant to James and me that day.

Angela's love for her job shows not only through her work but also through her compassion for patients and family members. She is truly exceptional. It is with great enthusiasm that I nominate her for recognition as one of this country's best oncology nurses! ❧

James Ott passed away in November 2013. We are proud to honor his memory.

The Power of Perseverance

BY ANGELA KRACH, RN, BSN

ANGELA KRACH, RN, BSN, has been a nurse at MD Anderson Cancer Center in Houston for 10 years. In that time, she has come to learn many things from her critically ill patients who are perpetually tethered to I.V. poles or confined to hospital beds. One of the biggest of those lessons is the power of perseverance.

"I SEE IT OVER and over again in this patient population," she says. "In what seems to me like a hopeless situation, a patient will say, 'I can get through this.' I've discovered the power of the body and the soul to persevere through it all."

She applies this lesson by passing along the sense of perseverance she gathers from one patient to inspire another.

That's exactly what happened with her patient James Ott, whose wife, Anne Falgoust Ott, wrote this year's winning essay. He was experiencing terrible complications from stem cell transplantation: graft-versus-host disease, encephalitis and pneumonia. When she had a one-on-one with him to assess what he thought of his situation, he surprised her.

"He just looked at me and said, 'I want to keep going. I want this for my friends. We can do this,'" Krach recalls. "And I was like, 'Yes, we can do this.'" Although Ott died in November 2013, she was able to utilize his sense of fortitude as she helped care for another very ill patient.

"He was severely ill and bleeding profusely," Krach says. Using Ott's words, she said to her patient, "We're going to do this."

"And he looked at me and said, 'Oh, absolutely.'" ✤

Advice From the Sky

FINALIST FOR THE 2013 EXTRAORDINARY HEALER AWARD FOR ONCOLOGY NURSING

STEVEN CUZZILLA, RN, ADN [VANDERBILT UNIVERSITY MEDICAL CENTER IN NASHVILLE, TENNESSEE]

WRITTEN BY CASSI JONES

MY HUSBAND and I first met Steven Cuzzilla when I was admitted to the hospital for a bone marrow transplantation. I'd been admitted at Vanderbilt several times before while undergoing chemotherapy, but we'd never had the pleasure of having Steven as our nurse. There were a select few night nurses that I always requested because, truthfully, I wanted to be able to sleep at night while in the hospital (and trust me, not all night-shift nurses are created equal). So I was a bit hesitant the night Steven walked through my door.

I KNEW he was a newer nurse, or so I had assumed, and I was unsure of how things would go. He came into the room at shift change, and I was pleasantly surprised. He was very thorough with his exam, asked a lot of questions and seemed genuinely interested in how I was feeling. Better yet, he was especially quiet during the night and worked by the glow of the computer screen, which meant I was able to sleep without being disturbed every two hours.

However, that's only the superficial part of what makes Steven such a wonderful nurse. I had Steven a couple of nights in a row, so we had the opportunity to talk and share our life stories. One night in particular my husband and I had been in deep discussion about our future and what decisions we should make concerning money, work and possibly relocating from our current home. Steven seemed to know I was extremely stressed out, because he took a seat at the end of my bed and just started talking to me. I told him all of my

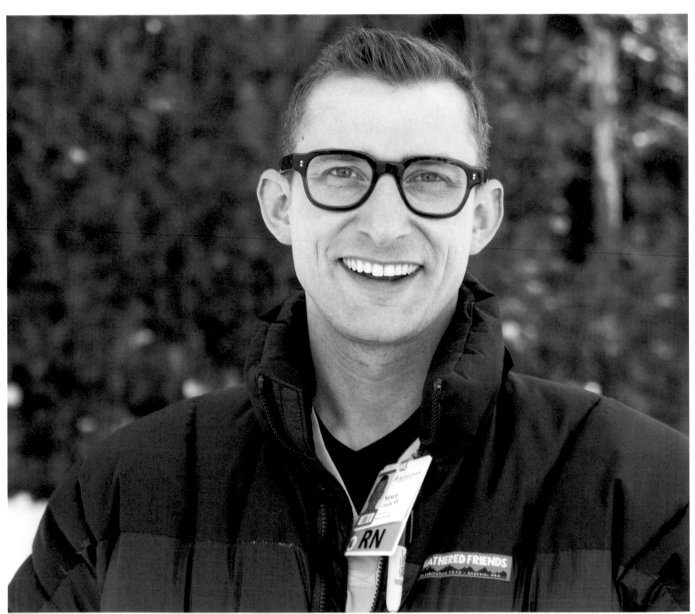

Steven Cuzzilla, RN, ADN

worries about work, money and life in general. This was when he took the time to share his story with me.

You see, Steven hasn't always been a nurse. This is his second career. He told my husband and me about his wife's diagnosis of cancer when she was in her 20s. I immediately glanced at his left hand because I was certain I didn't recall seeing a wedding band. His story continued, and he told us of his wife's battle with metastatic melanoma and her ultimate loss of that battle. It turns out that his wife was also treated at Vanderbilt University.

So, when he gave me advice about not worrying and trying to live in the moment, he was speaking from true experience. This had been his reality. He told us about how he and his wife never took anything for granted and that the only thing I needed to focus on was beating this cancer. He said to take each day as it came and not to focus on things years down the road because you never know when your last day will arrive. He wasn't being cynical; he was being honest and speaking from experience.

We really don't know when our last day will be, especially as a cancer patient, and most especially as a transplantation patient. He said that my husband and I should focus on us, on being together, on truly living each day and not just floating from one minute to the next.

I remember crying—no, sobbing—because I just couldn't believe his story. He was such a bubbly, fun-loving, relaxed guy. I would have never guessed that he had endured losing a wife. And the thought that he had changed his career and returned to the place she had died just so he could give back and help others who were going through the same thing he and his wife had—that was just mind-blowing. I knew I wasn't strong enough to do that. But here he was, sitting on my bed with that big, Italian smile and those brown, curly locks, and he was giving me advice. He was helping me, just as he had set out to do when he decided to change his career to oncology nursing.

He gave me the best advice I have ever received. He told me that any decision I made was the right one because at least I was making a decision. I shouldn't sit and worry about the consequences or if it was the "right" thing to do.

He then left me with his words of wisdom from a Lewis Carroll novel: "Every hole you jump in has a Jabberwocky in it, Alice, and you just have to keep going." It may seem simple, but when you are going through cancer, every decision is a hard one. You are facing life and death at the same time, and you fear that any decision you make will be the wrong one. You have so many regrets, so many wishes, and you just can't decipher what you should do. So, hearing Steven tell me to live out my life, do what I want, live life how it is supposed to be lived and enjoy it—that was what touched my heart. He had lived through those same fears and had those same thoughts, and he was paying it forward.

Our conversation ended shortly after that because he had to go hang chemotherapy in another room, and he'd already spent more than 40 minutes talking with me. But I will never, ever forget his words and advice. I will always try to live life as he described it to me, and I will never fear the "Jabberwocky" that appears in my route. I am forever indebted to Steven for his compassion, his willingness to take time out for me, his knowledge and skill as a nurse and, most of all, his determination to help us cancer patients. He has left a footprint on my heart and will never be forgotten. ❧

TEACHING MOMENT:

He gave me the best advice I have ever received. He told me that any decision I made was the right one because at least I was making a decision. I shouldn't sit and worry about the consequences or if it was the "right" thing to do.

The Power of Positivity

BY STEVEN CUZZILLA, RN, ADN

STEVEN CUZZILLA, RN, ADN, is still relatively new to the field of nursing.

"I'M SURE the things I have learned from patients most nurses have probably already experienced," he says. But his role as a bedside nurse allows him to spend lengthy stretches with patients, and from that time, he's absorbed important life lessons, one of the biggest being the power of positivity.

"I had this really great patient one time, and she had a note on her door that said 'No Frowning,'" Cuzzilla recalls. "I talked to her about it, and she said, 'Look, I don't want anybody in here that's going to be negative about this. If I have to live it, I want to live it the way I choose to live it.' I thought that was a really radical way of dealing with cancer."

Cuzzilla says this mantra of positivity can be applied to other challenging situations in life. For nurses, he says, one such challenge could be the current upheaval in health care.

"We're experiencing a lot of change right now, both at Vanderbilt and health care as a whole, and I think it's important for us to be positive about it," he says. "Yes, things are changing, but we don't have to go through it in a negative way. We can really dig out some good things about it."

On a smaller scale, he says that simply smiling can impact a person's life in a big way.

"What's really interesting is that the more you smile, the happier you seem to be, and then the people around you seem to smile a little bit more," Cuzzilla says. "Our attitude has a big influence on what life we lead." ❧

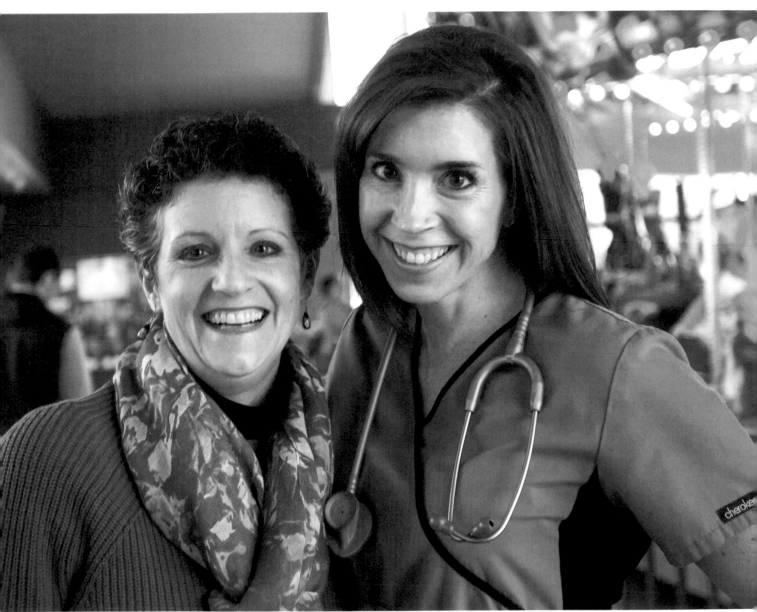

Julie Hinson, RN, BSN, OCN, with Joyce Lowry [left]

She Held My Hand Across the World

FINALIST FOR THE 2013 EXTRAORDINARY HEALER AWARD FOR ONCOLOGY NURSING

JULIE HINSON, RN, BSN, OCN [SALEM CANCER INSTITUTE IN SALEM, OREGON]

WRITTEN BY JOYCE LOWRY

CANCER ENTERS our lives unbidden and sometimes stubbornly refuses to leave. The journey we take from diagnosis onward is different for everyone. This unpredictable trail is filled with arduous climbs, zip-line descents and crazy hairpin turns. Having a special nurse to guide you along the way is a gift beyond compare.

I MET JULIE HINSON in November 2010, when I was referred to Dr. Elizabeth Munro after having developed an unusual vaginal discharge 10 years post–cervical cancer. Julie's cheerful demeanor easily drew me in, and I instantly felt I was in very good hands. Over the past few years, we have shared some very difficult moments as well as many instances of joy. She can help me see the humor in situations that seem as far from joy as can be imagined. I am so blessed to have gone through the past few months with her at my side.

Although I did not have cancer at that time, Dr. Munro and Julie kept close tabs on me, with frequent follow-ups to ensure that all was well.

Julie's joy was palpable when, in December 2011, I told her I was moving to Okinawa, Japan, to work on one of our U.S. air bases. It was to be the adventure of a lifetime. We kept in touch for the first six months of my journey. Weekly updates filled her in on all I was experiencing in a new culture.

I returned to the States for the summer months and, of course, had my routine follow-up exam with Dr. Munro. I had been back on Okinawa just three days when Dr. Munro called to tell me I had tested positive for cancer. I was stunned. Ten years after cervical cancer… it doesn't typically return. But here it was, and I was half a world away. A check with the U.S. Naval Hospital on Okinawa revealed that there were no gynecologic oncologists there and that I would need to return to the U.S. for treatment. Julie jumped into action completing the various documents the federal government needed in order to write my travel orders and put me on a flight to Oregon. Julie didn't hesitate when documents needed to be filled out, scanned and sent. She worked so hard to get everything done. In the middle of all this, Typhoon Bolaven, a category 4 storm, hit the island of Okinawa. Throughout the storm, Julie was on the phone and email, helping me work through necessary documents and assuring me I would soon be on my way.

Upon my arrival in the United States, Julie was there to greet me with a warm hug and her ever-present cheerfulness. She had my scans and surgery arranged and knew me well enough to know I like lots of information. Dr. Munro works out of two different hospitals in two separate cities. Because my surgery was to be robotic, it was scheduled at the larger facility, not the one where Julie worked. Nevertheless, I wasn't off her mind. She sent messages letting me know she was thinking of and praying for me and that she knew I was in the best hands.

I traveled the months of chemotherapy with Julie by my side. When side effects seemed insurmountable, Julie was there by phone or email to see me through. On the days that I struggled, though I lived an hour from the hospital, I felt Julie's presence. Her compassion infused with humor was the perfect prescription.

Upon completion of treatment, it was time to get back to Okinawa and back to work. Julie again spent endless hours filling out government documents so that I could receive travel orders for my return. One Friday evening at 5:30, Julie sent me a document that she had spent hours completing. When I received it, I realized it was not the document I needed. I had sent her the wrong one. When Julie learned this, she cheerfully asked me to send the correct one and said she would start right in on it. Keep in mind that Julie has a young family and is working on her master's degree; the last thing she needed was a new document at 5:30 on a Friday evening. Yet there was no hesitation or frustration on her part, just her usual cheerfulness.

I have just returned to Okinawa. As it should be, I am adjusting to walking this journey of health without Julie at my side. I am comforted, however, by knowing she will always be there when I need her to hold my hand across the world. ❧

The Power of Presence

BY JULIE HINSON, RN, BSN, OCN

JULIE HINSON, RN, BSN, OCN, has spent most of her seven years of nursing in the oncology ward. Along the way, many have asked about her choice of career. "They say, 'Oh, that's got to be hard. How do you do it?'" she says. "But I view nursing as a gift. We get to know people at probably one of the most intimate times in their lives, and it is a privilege to be allowed into their inner circle."

HINSON SAYS SHE has learned many things from her patients. Because they are often faced with uncertain futures, they see life from a unique perspective.

"They teach me how to be a better caregiver and a better nurse," she says, "and the way they do that is they have a super-clear outlook on their lives. They realize what is valuable and what is not."

Her patients have also taught her about the power of being physically present, especially when someone is going through a difficult time.

"I don't always have to have the right words or the right intervention," Hinson says. "I've learned how valuable it is to just be with them in the midst of their highs and lows and the whole emotional terrain that goes along with a cancer diagnosis." She does this by simply sitting in patients' rooms, listening to them talk about their worries and fears, or putting her arm around them in times both challenging and celebratory.

"And I've tried applying this lesson to other areas of my life," she says, "knowing how important it is to just physically be there for someone." ✤

CHAPTER 1
Above & Beyond

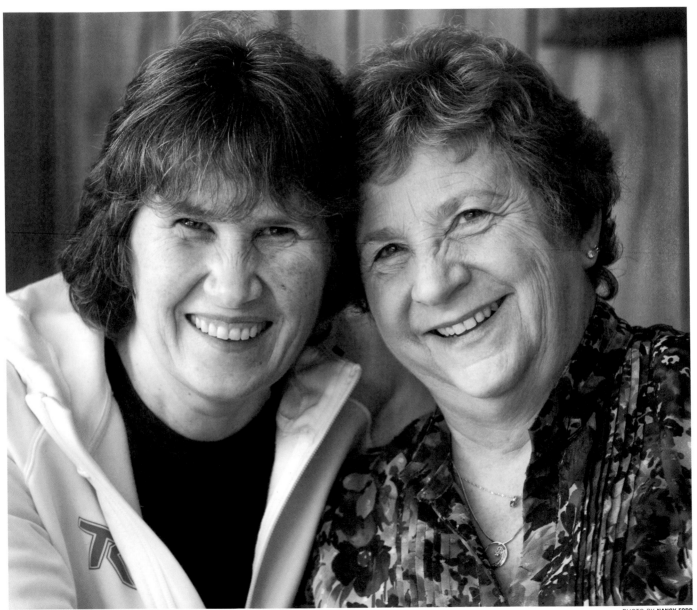

Karen Litwak, RN, ANP, APRN, AOCN, with Patti McGee [right]

Nurse, Caregiver, Ambassador and Friend

KAREN LITWAK, RN, ANP, APRN, AOCN [SUNY UPSTATE REGIONAL ONCOLOGY OFFICE IN ONEIDA, NEW YORK]   WRITTEN BY PATTI McGEE

IN MARCH 2003, at age 39, I received a diagnosis of estrogen-positive breast cancer. I was introduced to my oncologist and nurse practitioner at my first appointment. At that time, I didn't know how instrumental my nurse practitioner, Karen Litwak, would become to me during my treatment and for many years later.

DUE TO MY AGE, the oncologist wanted to treat my cancer aggressively every other week for 16 weeks. I would become violently ill for the first 72 hours after each of the first four treatments. I would contact Karen, and she would have me come in for I.V. fluids or blood work. After the third treatment, I became extremely ill. I developed eye infections, a chest infection and a rash up my right arm. Karen would always take my phone calls and see me immediately, regardless of the time of day.

But my journey with Karen really began when I started my post-cancer treatment regimen of drugs. I was scheduled to take a hormone therapy drug for five years, beginning in September 2003. About the third month in, right before Thanksgiving, I remember calling Karen. I was crying hysterically, eating a box of cupcakes in front of my refrigerator and wondering what was wrong with me. I couldn't stop crying. Karen told me to stop taking the drug and wanted to know if I was suicidal. I told her I wasn't, but I just couldn't stop crying. She explained to me that it was a side effect of the hormone therapy drug, and she would talk to the oncologist to see what we should do.

She returned my call the next day, and we set forth a plan for me to wait a few months and then try again. Throughout my journey, I experienced many side effects of the post-cancer drugs. Most were very debilitating and made me depressed. In December 2003, Karen recognized not only my struggles with cancer, but those of other patients and joined me in forming the Oneida Area Cancer Support Group. We co-chair the monthly support group, as well as an I Can Cope educational series through the American Cancer Society. It is still going strong 10 years later.

In 2004, Karen and I formed the Oneida Area Relay for Life, which we co-chaired until 2007. We brought in more than $750,000 to the area. Karen took on the role of survivor chair at the relay and enrolled more than 300 survivors, providing much-needed emotional support and hope for us. In 2005, we offered a Cancer Prevention Study 3 at our relay, and Karen recruited more than 300 participants as the chairperson. To this day, we still hold the record for most participants in the New York/New Jersey region of the American Cancer Society. In 2006, Karen and I were selected to be ambassadors for the American Cancer Society. We traveled to Washington, D.C., where we lobbied Congress for more cancer research funding in the New York state budget. Karen was also instrumental in securing funding for two other survivors to attend with us.

Over the past 10 years, I have witnessed Karen as she fights to get patients into clinical trials, comforts families when a patient's battle has ended and reassures us survivors that life will get better if we take it one day at a time. You'll find Karen staying after work to return phone calls, to seek funding for treatments and to do research for a patient. Karen gives all of us cancer survivors the hope to keep fighting and encourages us to be proactive. She feels that if you are involved in the decision-making process about your treatments, you will tolerate them better.

The thing I love most about Karen is her honesty with her patients. She is frank and open with them, regardless of the outcome of their diagnoses. She is there for them right to the end. I believe part of Karen's compassion comes from her experience as a caregiver. Karen's husband, Paul, is a prostate cancer survivor, and she has been there every step of the way for him. She has been a stabilizing force for me and the oncology community in our area. We are fortunate to have her as an oncology nurse practitioner.

In my darkest moments, when I felt like I couldn't go through one more round of chemotherapy or I was so depressed and didn't know who I was in the following years, Karen Litwak was there, providing me with hope and compassion to win this battle against cancer. She has dedicated her life to helping others through being a nurse, first, as well as a caregiver, an ambassador and, mostly, a friend. I am so blessed to have gotten breast cancer, because it brought Karen into my life. ❧

Lisa Is Taking Care of It

LISA ARMAO, RN, FNP, ANP-C [WOMEN'S CANCER CARE ASSOCIATES IN ALBANY, NEW YORK]

WRITTEN BY KELLY QUIST-DEMARS

"KELLY, IT'S LISA. Your file just came across my desk. Why didn't you call me?" I stammered out something about not knowing exactly where she worked and not being able to think clearly in general. Lisa had been married to my Uncle Bob while I was in my 20s, but they'd since parted ways.

Above & Beyond

FROM THE BEGINNING, Lisa became a part of our family, fitting in as if she had always been there. I knew she worked with women with cancer, but to me that meant breast cancer. While I didn't know where she worked, I knew she was tremendously dedicated to her patients.

A wave of relief passed through me when she said, "I have your file. I'm taking over; I will get you through this." I immediately called my mother, completely choked up with tears of relief, fear and other emotions I'd been holding inside. I had received a diagnosis of ovarian cancer just a month before, at the age of 30. We both felt lost and confused, knowing nothing about this type of disease. On the phone with my mother that day, I couldn't say much but managed to get out, "Lisa called. She is going to take care of me." That was all that needed to be said.

From that point on, we knew I had a staunch advocate and a compassionate professional on my side. Lisa was going to take care of it. "Lisa is taking care of it" is a common phrase at Women's Cancer Care Associates in Albany, New York. You hear it in the waiting room, the chemo room and the exam room.

As a nurse practitioner, Lisa is able to listen and be on the front lines. She can make treatment decisions that will immediately ease a patient's mind and her symptoms. It is easy to think that I got special treatment because Lisa is a family member, but to Lisa, everyone is family. "Lisa is taking care of it" for everyone.

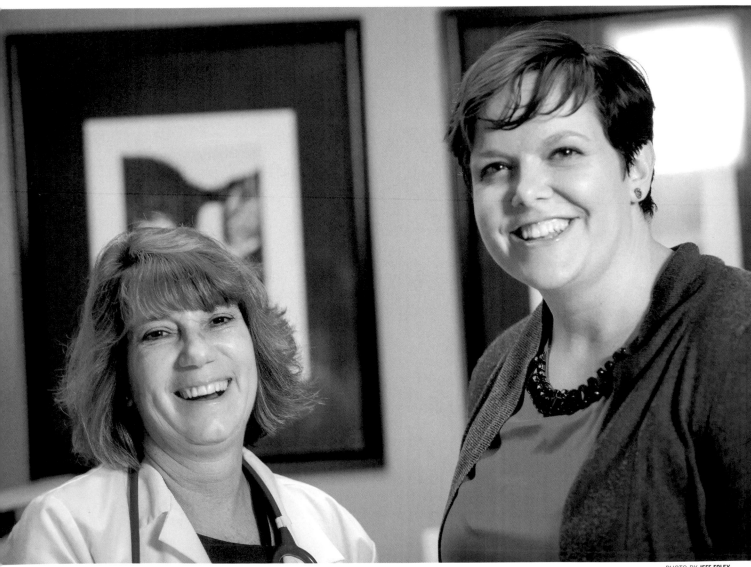

Lisa Armao, RN, FNP, ANP-C, with Kelly Quist-Demars [right]

In fact, most cancer patients have a team of caregivers and loved ones ready to support them. Lisa never acts as if the extra family members are a burden or taking up space. Lisa includes them in the conversations and decision-making. She takes the time to discuss everyone's concerns and tailors her approach to each individual. At my first chemo session, a man supporting the woman in the chair next to me commented, "Lisa always remembers my name. While I know it's not about me, it's just nice to be noticed." An experienced oncology nurse has seen and heard it all; a wise oncology nurse treats each patient with the understanding that this is the first time that she is going through it. Lisa has mastered this wisdom. She never brushed off my concerns.

This was especially true one weekend when I tried to self-diagnose a rash. So as not to bother Lisa on her day off, I figured I could solve the problem myself by looking at pictures of rashes on the Internet. After choosing the picture that best represented what I thought I had, I quickly realized it was serious and I should let Lisa know. Around 10 a.m. on a Saturday, I sent Lisa a text stating I had plaque psoriasis. Instead of telling me how incredibly unlikely that was, she simply replied, "Why do you think that?" She didn't judge and, more importantly, didn't disregard my symptoms. She walked me through it and together we determined that a switch in laundry detergent while my body was so susceptible to allergic reactions was what did it. A round of steroids, some hydrocortisone and a ton of laundry fixed the problem. My skin cleared up and I was left with my pride intact, feeling I was acknowledged as a person and not as an inconvenience with an annoying habit of self-diagnosing.

When life became a series of tests, appointments, opinions and words I didn't understand, knowing that Lisa was there to listen, to explain things to me and to acknowledge my individual spirit meant the world. Lisa is taking care of it.

When a person has cancer, "it" encompasses so many things. "It" is the patient's cancer—the side effects, the blood work, the endless medical tests. "It" is the patient's emotional state—the worries, the fears, the helplessness. "It" is the patient's family, friends and network. Lisa takes care of it all. As a dedicated healer, a staunch advocate and a compassionate professional, Lisa is taking care of it. ❧

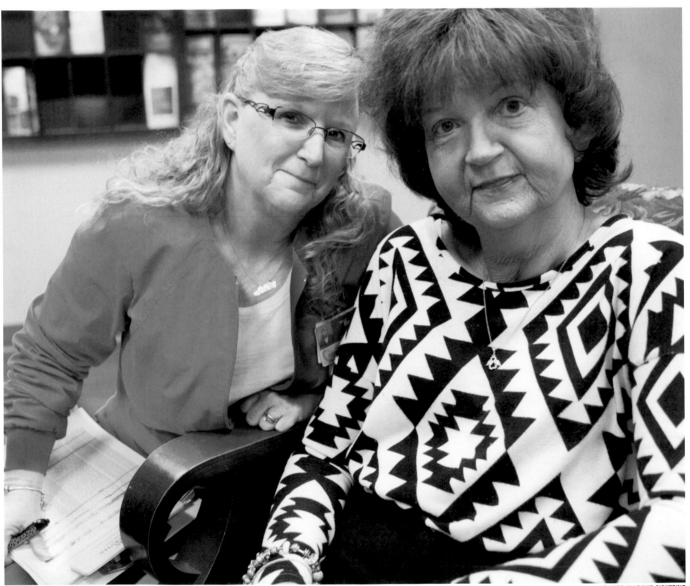

Barbara Gregory, RN, OCN, with Kathy D. Scott [right]

PHOTO BY DAVID PICKERING

A Nurse's Persistence

BARBARA GREGORY, RN, OCN [AUDRAIN MEDICAL CENTER AT SSM HEALTH CARE IN MEXICO, MISSOURI]
WRITTEN BY KATHY D. SCOTT

I AM AN 18-YEAR survivor of breast cancer.

I ORIGINALLY received a diagnosis of stage 2 disease in my right breast in 1995, at the age of 39. I began seeing Dr. Shahid Waheed for chemotherapy treatment after my mastectomy. Barbara Gregory was the oncology nurse who administered my chemo. Right from the start, I felt so comfortable with her. She would explain everything thoroughly before giving me a drug.

She was caring, compassionate and made me feel as if I was her number one priority. I felt she took a genuine interest in me as a person dealing with cancer, not as just another patient she had to tend to that day.

I made it through my six-month treatment regimen and then began follow-up visits. Every time I was in the office, I felt Barb was truly interested in my well-being. As months turned to years, I was finally down to annual checkups. Although I was always a little nervous at these visits, I always received good news. At the five-year mark, I finally started feeling more confident that the cancer would not return. After all, aren't you considered "cured" after the five-year cancer-free milestone?

Feeling more comfortable with my situation, I began postponing my annual checkups. I was feeling excellent, I had no symptoms and I was a very busy working wife and mother of three. I felt I had made it through the worst and come out on the other side by beating cancer. But every time I would go in for one of my annual checkups a few months late, Barb would always frown at me and let me know I really needed to make those visits a priority.

Fast-forward to my 10-year milestone. After nine years of cancer-free follow-up visits, I was not worried about my cancer returning, and I decided I did not need to go for any more checkups unless I noticed something wrong. It just seemed pointless to me to take time out of my busy schedule.

Around that time, I had ordered a new breast form and needed a prescription for it. I called Dr. Waheed's office and told them what I needed and that I would stop in one day on my lunch hour and pick it up. When I went in, I expected to just pick up the prescription out front from the receptionist, but Barb met me instead. She handed me the prescription and asked me why I was late with my annual checkup. I told her, "It's been over 10 years!" In response, I received a brief but serious lecture about how important my checkups were, no matter how many years had passed.

I went back to work feeling guilty, thinking about what she had said, so I picked up the phone and scheduled the appointment. I went in for the office visit, and they did the regular physical exam and lab work. A few days passed, and I received a phone call from Barb. She said there were some concerns about the results of my blood work. After more tests I received the devastating news that my cancer had returned and metastasized to my bones. I had been ignoring the bone pain I had recently noticed by telling myself I was just getting older or maybe it was arthritis. I attributed the severe pain in my left thigh bone to overdoing it on the treadmill.

TEACHING MOMENT:

I am 100 percent convinced that I would not be alive today if not for Barb. She cared enough to lecture me when I was so busy with everything else in my life that I was ignoring signs and symptoms.

Since receiving this news in 2005, my life has turned into rounds of chemotherapy and another mastectomy in 2011, when I developed a tumor in my other breast. The cancer has now spread to other parts of my body, including my throat and liver. But I am 100 percent convinced that I would not be alive today if not for Barb. She cared enough to lecture me when I was so busy with everything else in my life that I was ignoring signs and symptoms.

If she had not cared enough or taken the time on her lunch hour that day to talk to me, I would have continued burying my head in the sand until it would have been too late. Barb went above and beyond what was required. She is an outstanding nurse, and I am still here today fighting this fight because of her. ❧

I'll Be Home for Christmas

DONNA LaBARGE, RN, BSN, OCN [THE OHIO STATE UNIVERSITY WEXNER MEDICAL CENTER IN COLUMBUS, OHIO]   WRITTEN BY EMILY FLEMING

IT WAS DECEMBER 18, 2012, and my husband and I were driving the hour-long commute to the breast center at the Ohio State University Wexner Medical Center. I was to receive my fourth chemotherapy infusion since learning the breast cancer that was in my liver and bones had progressed and moved into my lungs. Less than 24 hours later, we'd make the same drive with our 3-year-old son to the Columbus airport to fly to San Diego for Christmas at "home" with my mom, dad, brother and sister.

CHRISTMAS AT HOME, surrounded by my family, was the most important thing to me during this most challenging time in my life. Though I didn't speak a word during this drive to my appointment, my mind was deep in conversation: *Okay… packing list is printed. I've laid out most of Bryce's stuff, and the laundry is done. The dogs are at the kennel. Now I just need my chemo … please, PLEASE let my neutrophils be up enough to get my chemo. Wow! Tomorrow is almost here! I'm actually going to make it home for Christmas! Uhhh … I can barely hold my head up … this chemo has beaten me to a pulp. Will this be my last Christmas? I can't fight the tears. I can't bear to leave Bryce without his mom. Will he remember what my love feels like? It's getting harder and harder to snap out of these dark moments. One thing at a time … chemo. God, I hope I am not dying.*

I took a deep breath as we walked out of the elevator onto the fourth floor of the breast center and to the receptionist's desk. With impeccable timing, Donna LaBarge walked toward the desk from the back and gave me a huge, heartfelt hug. "Donna! I am so glad to see you, too! Nope … not quite packed but at least

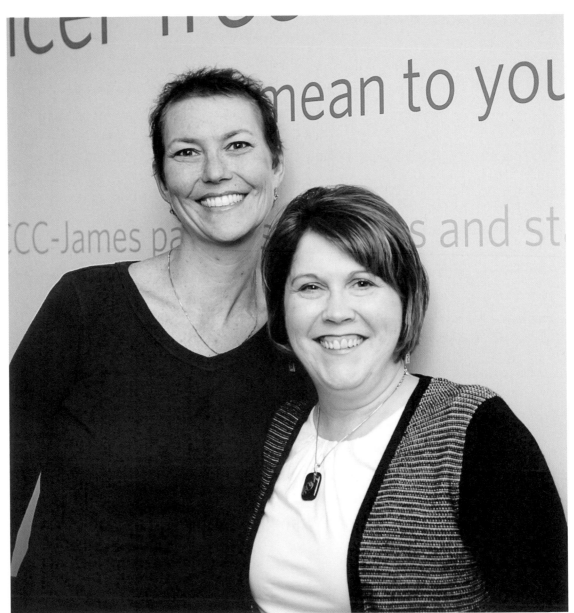

Donna LaBarge, RN, BSN, OCN, with Emily Fleming [left]

everything is organized. At 7 a.m., we're out of Columbus," I answer after being asked when we're leaving the next morning.

The darkness I'd allowed myself during the drive to Columbus melts away in Donna's company. I forget I have cancer. I feel like a normal person! Although she's only been Dr. Shapiro's nurse for about six months, I could swear I've known her for 15 years, like I'm in the company of an old friend. Since her arrival, my doctor visits feel like team efforts, and this enhances my confidence. Wait time is minimal and I still get the same, if not improved, Dr. Shapiro. Donna is a brilliant manager and a compassionate, talented nurse. She has helped me through so much. If she hasn't heard from me in a few days, she calls to see how I am doing. She's been concerned and encouraging. She answers questions and provides valuable advice.

I sit down in the waiting area smiling, suddenly proud of my cancer journey and myself. It's noon. In just a few hours, we'll be on our way home, and in 24 hours, we'll be close to landing in San Diego. Ahhh … I take a deep cleansing breath and smile some more. The chemo is so effective against breast cancer. My tumors must be shrinking away. Amazing how my perspective has suddenly changed. At the end of the appointment Donna and I hug again, and I'm reassured she cares about my family and me. "Have a great time, enjoy yourself and CALL ME anytime," she says. "You've got your oral chemotherapy for this cycle. I will take care of the preauthorization for the next cycle. You don't worry about it. Just have a good time with your family."

TEACHING MOMENT:

Donna is a brilliant manager and a compassionate, talented nurse. She has helped me through so much. If she hasn't heard from me in a few days, she calls to see how I am doing.

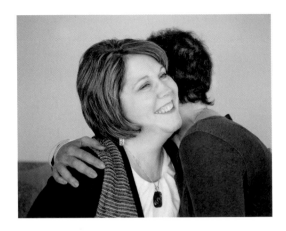

Dazed, my husband and I leave the deserted breast center. It is 8:30 p.m.

I'd had blood work, a chest X-ray, a CT scan and the expedited tumor markers assays. Most hadn't been scheduled prior to my arrival that day. Tests proved the chemo wasn't working. I worried our Christmas plans would dissolve. Donna had worked tirelessly, while still running Dr. Shapiro's service (which included seeing me three times instead of one), to ensure a comprehensive visit so Dr. Shapiro would have all the information he needed to decide whether to change my treatment. Both terrified and relieved that my last treatment was already off the list of strategies against my metastatic breast cancer, I was grateful that in just 10 short hours we'd be on a plane to San Diego. Christmas, perhaps my last, would be spent with my family at home, with no treatment delays or compromise. Wow, what a day.

Thank goodness for Donna. I can't imagine my cancer journey without her. Because of her, I feel safe. I think it really is going to be okay and that the new chemo *is* going to work. I will feel better, and I can't wait to tell her. She'll be so proud.

While I maintain hope that someday cancer will be a disease of the past, it has afforded me the privilege of knowing people such as Donna LaBarge. Because of her, my life is better and brighter. Because my life is better and brighter, my family will be okay. This I know, and so I smile and look forward to next Christmas. ❧

All the Difference

ANN PUGLISI, RN, BSN, OCN [NORTHSHORE UNIVERSITY HEALTHSYSTEM KELLOGG CANCER CENTER IN EVANSTON, ILLINOIS] WRITTEN BY BARBARA D. WICK

"NURSES ARE THE ONES who can make the difference between a bad experience and a good one."

Above & Beyond

ANN PUGLISI not only said that, she lives it each day. I have benefited enormously from her care. As a longtime ovarian cancer patient (originally diagnosed in mid-2003, I am now being treated for my fifth recurrence), I have had many experiences with nurses. Most are caring, patient, attentive people. Ann is that and more.

We met in 2008, when she joined my gynecological oncologist's team as his collaborative nurse. Because I can't seem to stay out of treatment for very long, we have typically been in contact at least once a week for almost five years.

While caring for patients with hematologic malignancies, Ann realized that oncology was her calling and earned her chemotherapy and biotherapy certifications. After a short time at Northwestern Memorial Hospital, she discovered she missed oncology, so she joined Kellogg Cancer Center, where I am a patient.

Part of what makes Ann special is her commitment to me. She engages me, and ensures that I get what I want and need to understand. She relates to me on a personal level and truly feels my issues, my ups and downs, my fears and hopes, and seeks solutions for each. Ann sees herself as my advocate and a partner in my struggle, especially when I am going through a tough time.

I have been reminded of Ann's advocacy in myriad ways. For example, she made sure that it was okay for me to have dental work; she checked with the pharmacologists and oncologist that the drug being recommended to tackle precancerous skin cells on my face would not interfere with my treatment drugs; and she recommended another drug "add-on" to kick my treatments to a more effective level.

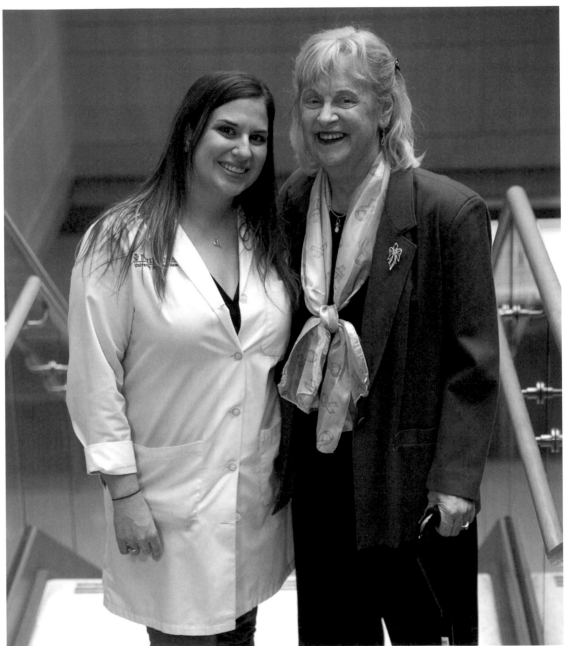

Ann Puglisi, RN, BSN, OCN, with Barbara D. Wick [right]

I faced some exceptionally rough times getting one particular chemotherapy drug. I am very allergic to the stuff, yet through consultation with the doctor and the pharmacologist, Ann was convinced they could get me through, using a combination of steroids, antihistamines and timed treatments—not to mention some positive mental attitude, imaging and personal attention.

To reduce the risk, Ann situated me in a room across the hall from her desk so she could keep an eye on me and detect early signs of an allergic reaction. We settled in for an extended series of long days together. Often she'd sit with me or make sure someone else was there. It was hairy at times, and yet we had many moments of warmth and laughter. Her calm and cheerful focus gave me the courage to move ahead and the confidence to face each treatment and its risks. She got me through.

Ann likes to learn and appreciates it when I read and share an article on an upcoming treatment, trial result or possible use of a supplement. She uses what she learns to find creative new solutions to my issues and dreams with me of prevention and cure. Because I like coaching, she helps me interact with other patients.

Ann finds ways to build up my relationship with my doctor by providing shared experiences outside

TEACHING MOMENT:

Ann likes to learn and appreciates it when I read and share an article on an upcoming treatment, trial result or possible use of a supplement. She uses what she learns to find creative new solutions to my issues and dreams with me of prevention and cure.

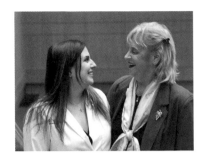

of treatment. One way is by becoming the organizer for her unit's team, Team Go, for the annual National Ovarian Cancer Coalition walk in Chicago. Each year she encourages us to join with our family and friends, creates a cute identifying item for us, persuades the physicians to join the team and cheers for us on the day of the walk. The funds raised and numbers involved are huge.

Ann is quite imaginative in finding ways to help me handle my unique array of side effects from my current treatment. That includes finding ways to reduce rashes and skin irritation; to drive away mouth sores; to keep my feet functional when faced with skin irritation and neuropathy; and to manage fatigue. While she does not harangue, Ann does, in her ever-cheerful and upbeat manner, check what is going on, what is working, what needs to be changed, and then persuades me to do it.

Compassion is critical, especially in the world of an ovarian cancer patient. So many of us will end our journeys in death from this disease. When my test results take a twist in the wrong direction, I can hear the pain in her voice. When they change for the better, even just a bit, she cheers me. This is not a mechanical response but true caring. Knowing the torture that waiting can be, Ann is assertive about getting results to me. She tracks answers down when they don't appear on time. She helps me prepare for my appointment with my oncologist, so I do not panic when we meet face to face. Ann gives me hope, and when the time comes, Ann will have the courage to stay close to me as I end my physical journey.

As my husband said, Ann became a girlfriend without impinging on a professional relationship. Her balance of pragmatism and compassion is reflected in the care she provides. Ann gets me through and is the difference in my cancer journey. ❧

As Strong as Steel

SANDRA STEEL, RN, BSN [DARTMOUTH-HITCHCOCK NORRIS COTTON CANCER CENTER IN LEBANON, NEW HAMPSHIRE]   WRITTEN BY PETER SMITH

AS HER NAME IMPLIES, Sandy is as strong as steel when it comes to navigating the medical and oncology world to be sure that her patients get the appropriate attention.

I MET SANDY soon after my surgery to remove a stage 4 glioblastoma multiforme brain tumor. Her role as a trial nurse in the clinical trial I had joined meant that she would be working closely with me to assure we were in full compliance with the rules. I quickly found out that the drug company subsidiary we had was from one of the biggest health insurers in the industry. It was constantly late in handling chemo prescriptions and was not acting in a professional manner. Sandy found out how this affected my stress level and tried to straighten out the problem, which was much bigger than a solo cancer-stricken patient new to the system could handle. In short, Sandy made my problems her problems. She kept one or two steps ahead of the drug company and contacted it to correct its errors in time to deliver the prescription.

We stayed in close contact this past year. I'm sure she secretly dreaded my calls but she didn't show it and virtually nothing escaped the net she had cast between herself and me. One other important fact to mention is that she is also a surviving cancer patient and found the energy and time to address my problems as well as those of other patients. Just seeing her with her hair covering was an inspiration to me. I thought, "If she can get through her cancer, a busy day and keep that up indefinitely, I am encouraged."

Dr. Fadul, who is in charge of my case, has let me know several times how he values Sandy's help with patients, too. As valuable as Sandy is, her ability to serve patients could be limited if not for team members such as Dr. Fadul and for the patient-centered measures that ease the burdens of patients and families at

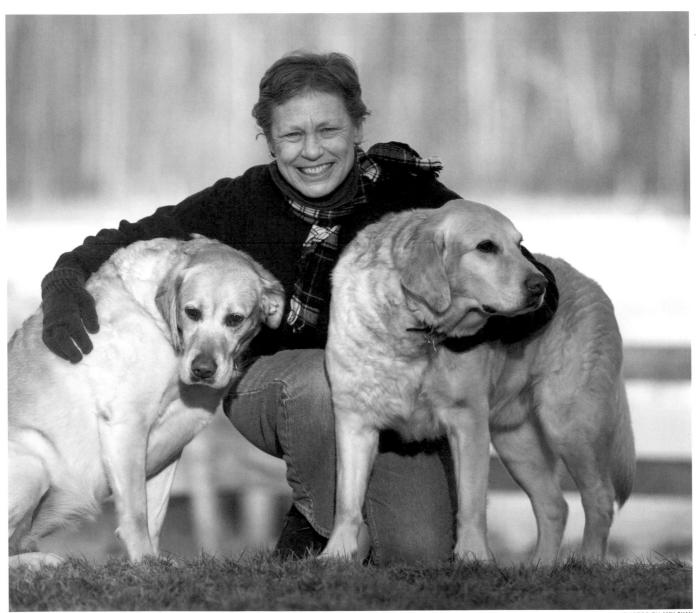

Sandra Steel, RN, BSN

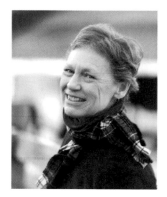

Dartmouth-Hitchcock. These measures include providing sandwiches and snacks during chemo in the infusion room, playing soothing music such as harp and piano in public areas and offering morning newspapers as well as creative writing and "ethical will" writing classes, all of which can help patients grow in some way and not just survive cancer treatments. Sandy's personal touch and these other supports add up to an amazing feeling of being cured and cared for. ❧

Peter Smith passed away in July 2013. We are proud to honor his memory.

TEACHING MOMENT:

Sandy made my problems her problems. She kept one or two steps ahead of the drug company and contacted it to correct its errors in time to deliver the prescription.

CHAPTER 2
Peer Tribute

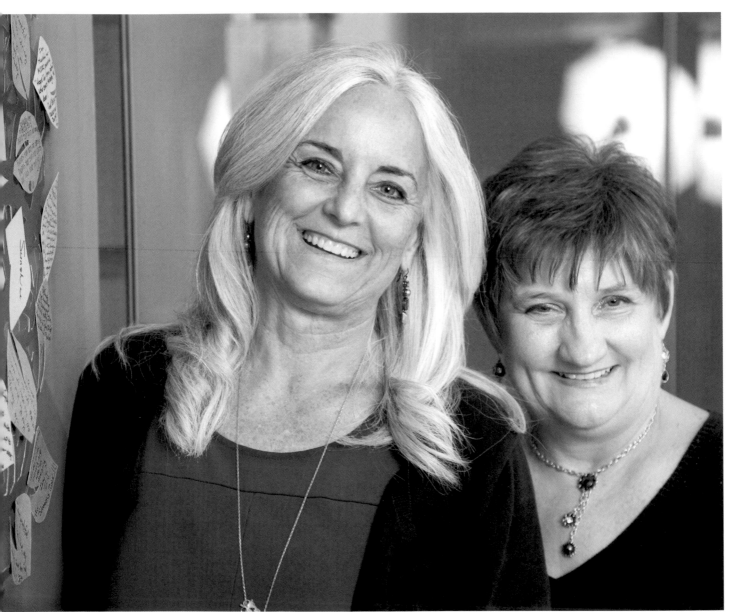

Cynthia Bedell, RN, MSN, NP-C, with Wanda Strange, RN, OCN [right]

Ordinary Days in the Life of an Extraordinary Nurse

CYNTHIA BEDELL, RN, MSN, NP-C [MARY CROWLEY CANCER RESEARCH CENTERS IN DALLAS]

WRITTEN BY WANDA STRANGE, RN, OCN

CYNTHIA BEDELL begins each day with an early morning run to maintain physical and emotional health. She arrives at the clinic by 7 a.m., ready to greet the first patient. From the first exam of the morning to the last phone call of the evening, every action centers on the patients. Pity anyone who mistreats or disrespects a patient under her care.

A TIRELESS ADVOCATE, Cindi works hard to ensure all patients receive the care they deserve. Here are a few glimpses into the days of this extraordinary nurse practitioner.

A gentleman fidgets in the bed of the procedure room as he waits. While staff members provide necessary details, the patient remains extremely apprehensive. Cindi calmly explains each step before it happens, easing the anxiety of the patient and his wife. Reflecting on the experience, the patient says, "It wasn't nearly as bad as I anticipated. I should have realized it would be okay. Everything [Cindi] told me has been right so far."

Always quick to participate in anything that brings a smile to the faces of the patients, families and staff, Cindi never misses an opportunity to celebrate life and make each person feel special. Her unique sense of humor brings a much-needed lightness to a serious atmosphere. A good report results in Cindi's performing a Snoopy "happy dance." Everyone shares the moment of joy with high fives and hugs. Often, treatment regimens make birthday celebrations in the clinic a necessity. Cindi purchases, decorates and presents a box containing a cupcake as she leads the staff in a birthday serenade.

"One of the ways Cindi shines brightest is when patients are given bad news," says a long-time co-worker. "The natural tendency is to pull away because we don't know what to say. Cindi reminds me of the haunting photos of heroic firefighters charging into a burning building to rescue and aid terrified victims. That's the Cindi I admire most, running to comfort patients and families when it is the most uncomfortable thing to do. Extraordinary!"

One patient initially refused to be examined by anyone but a doctor. However, within a few short weeks, she refused to see anyone but Cindi. Another woman, who had recently lost her father, sought out Cindi, whom she had met only once, to ask how she could help other patients. Cindi takes a young widow to dinner to make sure she is okay. Patients often seek her out, even when they aren't scheduled to see her, just to feel reassured by her hug.

"I am realistic," one caregiver remarked, "but I feel so much more hopeful after talking to Cindi today."

She explains procedures thoroughly, easing the patients' anxiety. She breaks down complicated protocols so patients and caregivers understand clinical trials. Support groups love the way she presents complicated information so they understand.

Cindi's also been known to make house calls. One sweet widow recalled a visit made to her late husband: "He'd do things for Cindi that no one else could get him to do."

TEACHING MOMENT:

She explains procedures thoroughly, easing the patients' anxiety. She breaks down complicated protocols so patients and caregivers understand clinical trials.

While many of her counterparts are heading home to relax, Cindi volunteers her time educating or serving the community. She lectures oncology nurses about a new drug. On Wednesday evenings, she provides care to uninsured and indigent patients at a community clinic. She passionately pursues treatment and solutions for these patients with the same energy she gives all her patients.

In her free time, she can be found preparing documents for future teaching lectures or watching her daughter's sporting events. She spends hours at home reviewing charts of new patients, matching them to appropriate clinical trials. Often, she answers calls in the middle of the night, and, once awake, she meticulously records details to pass along to the staff the following day.

Before Thanksgiving dinner, Cindi sends text messages to families who recently lost loved ones, acknowledging their grief and loss.

A role model for colleagues, Cindi leads by example, modeling professionalism, compassion and tenderness. Her skills as an educator are outstanding. She co-authored several cutting-edge research papers with the team at Mary Crowley Cancer Research Centers. She frequently serves as a preceptor for nurse practitioner students. Challenging them to think through decisions, she encourages each student to achieve his or her personal best. She presents new drug information to oncology nurses in an interesting way that facilitates learning. Her inquisitive mind benefits her co-workers as she finds educational opportunities and encourages the staff to learn with her.

No matter how busy the day, she patiently explains, demonstrates and instructs. Her encouragement provides confidence to more reticent nurses to take on new challenges. A humble individual, Cindi would bristle at being described as extraordinary, I suspect.

In a recent leadership meeting, she articulated Mary Crowley's vision, which mirrors her own: Our mission is to deliver cutting-edge cancer therapies in the most compassionate way possible. Her co-workers are privileged to see Cindi at work as she provides excellent patient care, celebrates another patient's year of life, encourages patients with little hope and no reason to move forward to find hope, feel loved and know their lives have value.

We have all seen Cindi touched by our patients, whether through a smile, tears, a brief moment of silence to regroup or her determination to make sure that all her co-workers know the value of each and every life that walks through our door. Cindi inspires each of us to be passionate about what we do and how we treat our patients. She is loved by all and is most definitely an extraordinary healer. ❧

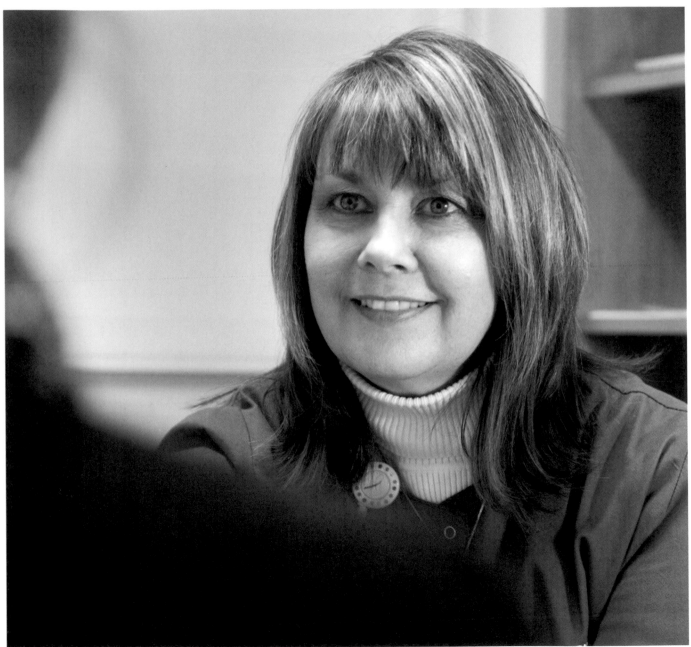

Jill Brown, RN, BSN, OCN, CBCN

A Bright Light in Darke County

JILL BROWN, RN, BSN, OCN, CBCN [WAYNE HEALTHCARE IN GREENVILLE, OHIO]

WRITTEN BY DANIEL P. McKELLAR, MD

IMAGINE LIVING in a small rural farming community and suddenly you find out you have cancer. What would you do? Who would you call? How would you find help and support? For patients living in Darke County, Ohio, these questions are now answered because they have a friend, neighbor and experienced oncology nurse they can turn to.

Peer Tribute

JILL BROWN has been an oncology nurse for more than 20 years. She has extensive experience providing chemotherapy as a navigator, home health nurse, clinical trials nurse and as an instructor in chemotherapy and biotherapy. Even though her talents and abilities would easily make her a candidate for a position in a larger cancer program, Jill has dedicated herself to caring for patients in the community where she and her husband live and farm. Unlike many oncology nurses, she doesn't focus on just one aspect of care for cancer patients.

Because Jill works in a small rural facility, she has to wear many hats to provide cancer patients with the care and support they need. Jill was responsible for helping establish the cancer program at Wayne HealthCare, including creating tumor boards, a cancer committee and a cancer registry, which helped us to receive accreditation by the Commission on Cancer in 2010 and to earn its prestigious Outstanding Achievement Award.

Jill was instrumental in starting an infusion center so patients did not have to make the 30-mile drive to a larger city to receive their chemotherapy. She is the clinical trials nurse, which means patients in this hospital have access to more than 60 National Cancer Institute clinical trials. Jill has found financial support for many cancer patients so they don't have to carry the burden of financial concerns while fighting their cancer. In addition, she has developed resources to provide a free mammogram to Darke County women who don't have insurance.

I could spend several pages writing about the many accomplishments Jill has made to help serve our cancer patients and to develop resources to allow them to receive high-quality care close to home. But it is what she provides to the patients on a one-to-one basis that is really important.

Every day, Jill gives compassionate support to patients by helping them with their emotional, physical and psychosocial needs. She is a friend, counselor, educator and sometimes just someone to provide a shoulder for patients to cry on or a hug to help them get through the day. Jill sees patients when they are diagnosed, before and after surgery, in the oncologist's office, in the infusion center, at the grocery store or even at the beauty salon. Jill rarely goes anywhere in the community without being recognized by a patient or family member, who often stops her to ask questions or provide an update. Jill always has a smile and a kind word for the patient or family member, but what she also always gives is time to address their needs.

In the short time since we started the cancer program at Wayne HealthCare, we have seen a tremendous increase in the number of patients who entrust us with their care. This type of reputation is not easy to establish, but through Jill's efforts in helping to bring all of the resources together, most importantly kind, compassionate support to patients, the community trusts that we will meet their needs.

I can't think of anyone more deserving of this award than Jill. She is truly passionate about oncology nursing and puts quality and safety at the forefront of her care. This passion shines through in her voice, her touch and her expressions as she interacts with patients, families and co-workers. She serves as a valuable clinical resource and inspires her peers to perform at their highest level, creating a culture of excellence within our cancer program. I truly appreciate Jill's hard work, talent and dedication to our community as she assists in making quality, patient-centered cancer care a reality in Darke County. ❧

A Nurse's Nurse

PAULINE BUSZKIEWICZ, RN [MASSACHUSETTS GENERAL HOSPITAL IN BOSTON]

WRITTEN BY LAURA LONG, RN, PhD

EVERY PATIENT remembers being told, "You have cancer." It is a watershed moment, replayed over and over; where I was, who I was with and how I felt. When I first heard the words "You have cancer," I was at work on a busy surgical floor at Massachusetts General Hospital. My job involves setting up home care services for patients, but suddenly I faced the new reality of being a patient. The news came in a phone call from my primary care physician, who went from telling me, "You have breast cancer," to providing phone numbers for a surgeon she recommended. The bustle and beeps of the hospital were replaced with swirling anxiety and uncertainty as I made cryptic notes about what she was saying, while the voice in my head kept saying, "You have cancer."

WITHOUT HESITATION, I walked upstairs to see Pauline Buszkiewicz. Pauline works as a case manager, coordinating discharge plans for patients going home after plastic and reconstructive surgery. Pauline knows what breast cancer surgery involves, but more importantly, she knows what being a cancer patient means.

Several years ago, Pauline faced her own battle with cancer; away from work for several months, she

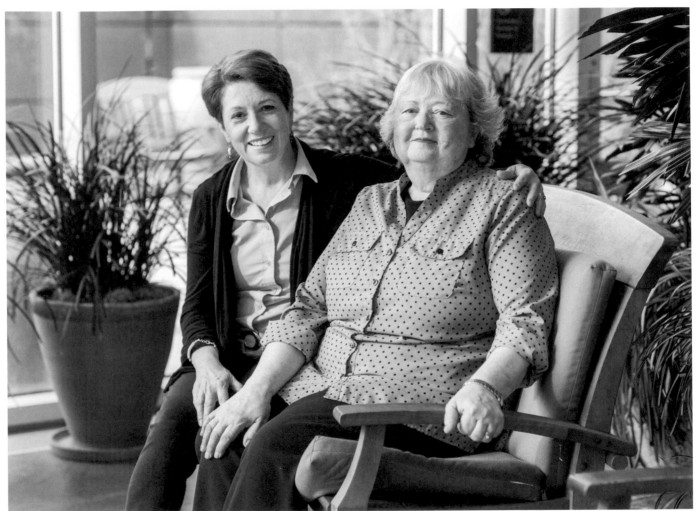

Pauline Buszkiewicz, RN, with Laura Long, RN, PhD [right]

returned after surgery and chemo. Her colleagues were initially struck by how different she looked, but more remarkable was the renewed energy and bright spirit Pauline brought back to work as a cancer survivor. Rather than focus on the negative, Pauline came back with a message about how fortunate she felt that her cancer had been diagnosed and treated at a wonderful institution like Mass General and how grateful she was to continue caring for others.

As I sat with Pauline and shared my news, she radiated empathy and compassion. She was able to say "I understand how you must be feeling" in ways none of my other work colleagues, family members or friends could. We talked about the difficult news and how unexpected it felt.

The voice in my head kept replaying those words "You have cancer." The words and meaning didn't seem to fit. They felt puzzling. Pauline understood the uncertainty. She let me focus on the feelings until I was ready to contemplate the options and decisions that lay ahead. Pauline helped me prepare for the reality that "you have cancer" is just the first of many layers of results to digest.

While I still couldn't believe that cancer was happening to me, the workup and results came incrementally, over the course of weeks. It did get worse; I had four tumors, and I had a relatively high risk of recurrence. Having a colleague like Pauline provided a gateway to knowledge about surgeons, treatments and choices. For me, Pauline was "a nurse's nurse."

TEACHING MOMENT:

Having a colleague like Pauline provided a gateway to knowledge about surgeons, treatments and choices. For me, Pauline was "a nurse's nurse."

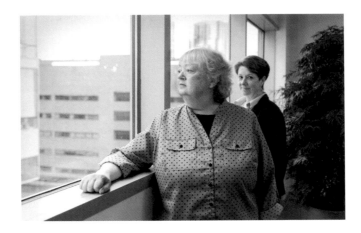

In the weeks leading up to my bilateral mastectomy and reconstructive surgery, I found it reassuring to be around Pauline, who was back to work and focused on caring for others. I decided to have a nipple-sparing mastectomy with immediate reconstruction using my own tissue, which meant a 10-hour surgery, scheduled on a Friday.

I didn't see Pauline until she returned to work the following Monday. It felt strange for me to be "the patient" in the Johnny gown, walking tentatively in the hallways, juggling drains. Pauline was there as a nurse, as a friend and as a cancer survivor. She made arrangements for my home care. Thanks in part to her coordination and expertise, I was able to leave the hospital in four days rather than five.

A few days after I was settled at home, I received a flower arrangement from the nurses on Bigelow 13, where I had been a patient. I knew Pauline was behind that unexpected expression of kindness. We corresponded through cards and my occasional visits after chemotherapy, which went on for six months.

I've now entered the longest phase of care, the "cancer survivor" phase. When I was in nursing school, patients like me were referred to as "cancer victims." Thankfully, cancer treatment has progressed. Although I haven't been able to return to work full time, I have been able to embrace Pauline's message. I feel fortunate that I came through the acute phase of cancer treatment at a hospital with excellent medical care, but more importantly, with caring nurses like Pauline. ❧

An Open-Door Policy

GAIL PROBST, RN, MS, ANP, AOCN, NE-BC [HUNTINGTON HOSPITAL IN HUNTINGTON, NEW YORK]
WRITTEN BY SUSAN SIMPSON, MSLIS

IT COMES … and it goes … and it comes … and it goes. This best describes my past 10 years as I've lived with metastatic colon cancer. My illness has developed a funny pattern, assuming you can call cancer funny. The disease presents itself, my practitioners rally and I get treated. I am then fortunate to hear "no evidence of disease" for two or three years until another recurrence, and the cycle repeats. Thankfully, my cancer does not hang around continuously, but the members of my healthcare team do.

GAIL PROBST is one of the many professionals who is part of Team Simpson. She has supported me during the past 10 years. I first met Gail in February 2003 when I received a diagnosis of metastatic colon cancer at the age of 39. Things were not looking so good those first few days. Gail and I spoke at length, and after she left my room, I felt more in control of a situation that was quickly spiraling out of control. She enhanced the game plan that had been previously discussed with my doctors and reinforced the hope that the practitioners initially gave me.

Gail continued to visit me every day before I was discharged from the hospital and instilled in me a sense of fight and peace at the same time. Thinking back to those difficult early days after that initial diagnosis, I can still clearly remember some of Gail's words of wisdom. She wisely suggested that I get second and third opinions and even made the arrangements for me to see another doctor at a larger cancer center. I asked Gail many, many questions, and she always returned my calls. Looking back, I can now see that some of them

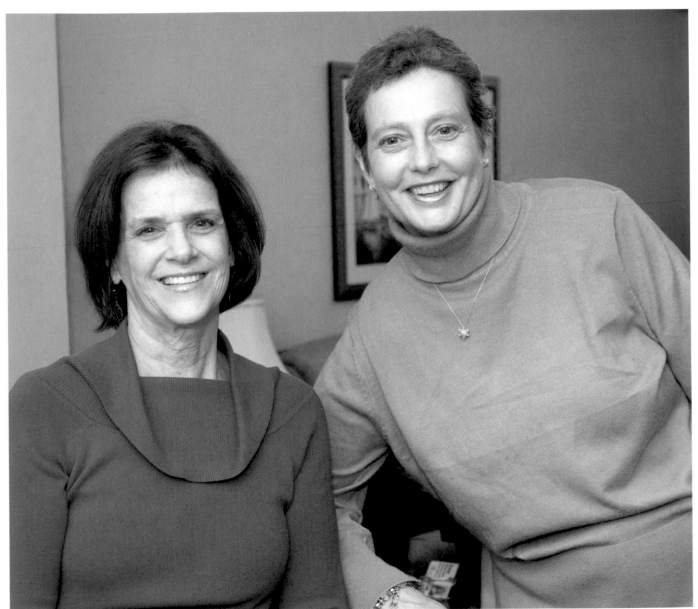

Gail Probst, RN, MS, ANP, AOCN, NE-BC, with Susan Simpson, MSLIS [right]

might have seemed a little silly: "Should I do yoga?" and "Is it okay to ask my doctors for sleep medication?" Gail never acted as if these were trite questions and always responded with a comforting answer.

I recently have had the misfortune of experiencing my fourth recurrence. A surveillance scan revealed tiny spots on my lungs and liver. I again have the privilege of being both a former and current patient of Gail's. I am also a co-worker of Gail's; we both work at the same community hospital.

Several years after I received my diagnosis, I decided to seek a different career, and after completing additional education, I was lucky enough to secure employment at Huntington Hospital. I now have the privilege of working with Gail and many other fine professionals who help make the world a better place. We have learned over the years that cancer is not one disease, but that there are probably hundreds of forms of primary cancer sources. The answers to questions regarding physical health can be difficult because of this. In addition, other variables add to the puzzle: Every treatment is different, and every person reacts to treatment differently. Gail clearly understands this and has the ability to react differently with her patients.

While Gail shares her infinite knowledge, she is quick to point out that sometimes there is no clear answer to every question. She helps her patients understand that there are often many courses of treatment for certain cancers. It is easier to be positive regarding my illness after listening to Gail rattle off the new drugs that are coming to market and the innovative ways that cancer is now being treated.

TEACHING MOMENT:

Thinking back to those difficult early days after that initial diagnosis, I can still clearly remember some of Gail's words of wisdom. She wisely suggested that I get second and third opinions and even made the arrangements for me to see another doctor at a larger cancer center.

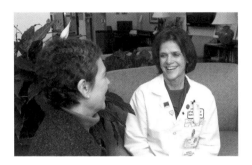

We survivors can be a difficult bunch. Some like to say they are cured, some prefer to be considered patients forever and others are somewhere between the two. Along with our current or lingering physical health issues, we also have emotional baggage. There is depression, anxiety, survival guilt and fear of recurrence, to name a few. Knowing the right thing to say and the appropriate way to approach a survivor can be tricky. Having taken care of probably hundreds of patients over the years, Gail has found the fine balance of knowing the right thing to say. Some years I insist that I am never done when it comes to cancer. Other times I am sending her journal articles that define the cure for my disease. Throughout the years, Gail will listen to what I have to say. She will then give both sides of the story. I always feel more grounded after leaving her office. She has helped support the theory that this is a chronic disease for me.

While Gail has helped me with both physical and emotional issues before, during and after my treatments, I am not her only patient. As director of cancer services at the hospital, Gail does this with dozens of patients each week. Her door is always open to patients, families and her co-workers. Gail is known as the go-to person in our hospital regarding cancer. Even employees who do not know Gail personally will ask to meet with her.

Once, I witnessed an employee gently knock on her door and say with hesitation, "Mary from Dietary said that it would be okay to come and talk to you about my daughter's cancer. I hope this is okay." Gail responded with a hearty welcome, dropped what she was doing and invited the employee into her office. I am proud to be a co-worker of Gail's because she always finds the time to speak with people who need her knowledge, expertise and empathy. With a grateful heart, I can say that Gail is an extraordinary healer. ❧

A Leader in the Field

DIANA TAM, RN, BSN, OCN [MEMORIAL SLOAN-KETTERING CANCER CENTER IN NEW YORK, NEW YORK]

WRITTEN BY ELIZABETH JOY, RN

DIANA TAM has worked at Memorial Sloan-Kettering Cancer Center for seven years, first in inpatient for two years and then in outpatient gastrointestinal cancer (GI) chemotherapy for five years. We have a clinical ladder system that recognizes and rewards those who have developed expertise in nursing practice. Diana has demonstrated leadership skills and now functions as a clinical nurse IV. She acts as charge nurse weekly, precepting new staff, and she employs strong interpersonal communication skills with both colleagues and patients; our unit is very lucky to have her! I have been an oncology nurse for 15 years and have been working in the outpatient setting at Sloan-Kettering on GI chemotherapy for the past three years. Since my employment here, Diana has stood out as a shining star.

Peer Tribute

WORKING IN OUTPATIENT, nurses see many patients on a consistent basis. Diana has developed a devoted fan base of those requesting her to be their nurse. She has expertise starting difficult I.V.s and exceptional skills managing complex chemotherapy and research protocol regimens. She has an extensive knowledge base of the GI disease process. She is full of energy and dedicated to delivering exceptional patient care.

In 2012, Diana received the DAISY Award from a nationwide program that celebrates the extraordinary clinical skill and compassionate care given by nurses. Numerous patients and co-workers made submissions on her behalf.

It is not surprising that Diana received this award, because her contributions to Sloan-Kettering are many. She has been a leader on behalf of GI chemotherapy to secure funds for nursing research and development through Sloan-Kettering's Geri and ME Fund. The fund provides ways for nurses to increase their skills and knowledge, all with the goal of improving the lives of cancer patients. Diana has also worked with another colleague to develop a peer-to-peer support group, an extension of our education lecture series. This series covers topics such as compassion, fatigue, burnout and resilience. In addition, she is the "wellness champion" for our employee wellness program and has organized our unit's weight-loss competitions. Diana also organized our unit's use of the Frederick Henry Prince IV Family Hospital Morale Program, which provides funding for projects that promote staff morale and team spirit. Finally, Diana led the effort to nominate the GI chemotherapy nurses for a nursing magazine's best nursing team award. Our unit came in second place.

Aside from these achievements, perhaps the story of Mr. F. will demonstrate how Diana embodies the characteristics of an extraordinary healer. She establishes a special connection with patients and families through trust and emotional support.

TEACHING MOMENT:

Diana has a talent for being able to find a special connection with a patient. For Mr. F., it has been through humor, and during his treatments, you can hear them laughing and enjoying each other's company.

It is neither a sad story nor one of great heroics, but a story of constancy and connection. Mr. F. received a diagnosis of colon cancer five years ago. He has been coming to our unit every two weeks, and Diana has administered the majority of his treatments. Over the course of those many months, they've forged a relationship, as Diana has listened, intervened and supported him as he lived his life with cancer. Mr. F. says he looks forward to his chemotherapy and connecting with "his" nurse, Diana. She appreciates and rejoices in the intimate details of his life, including the story of how he and his wife met on Fire Island, raised a family and recently married off his daughter and then his son; he has learned, he says, to be grateful for every day.

Diana has a talent for being able to find a special connection with a patient. For Mr. F., it has been through humor, and during his treatments, you can hear them laughing and enjoying each other's company. He struggles with comorbidities, along with his colorectal cancer. Diana has instructed him with regard to nutrition and lifestyle, and encouraged him to continue golfing. His wife has recently started a new job, so she will no longer be able to come with Mr. F. for his chemotherapy, but she told Diana that she feels comfort and assurance in knowing that he will be cared for by Diana.

Just recently, Mr. F. experienced a progression of his disease for the first time in five years. It is very scary for both him and his wife; together and separately they have discussed with Diana their fears and trepidations. After discussing his case with his oncologist, Diana blended hope with realism, focusing on what is in the present while preparing them for what may possibly be.

In summary, Diana has the unique ability to blend her professional knowledge and skills with compassion for those within her care. Through her assessment skills, she is always able to find that certain variable that connects her to the patient and family. Mr. F. could probably write a book about Diana, but, as he says, "Diana has made all the difference for me and my wife … And if you could say my chemotherapy was enjoyable, well, she has made it so, and I am so very grateful to her. She is simply the best!" ❧

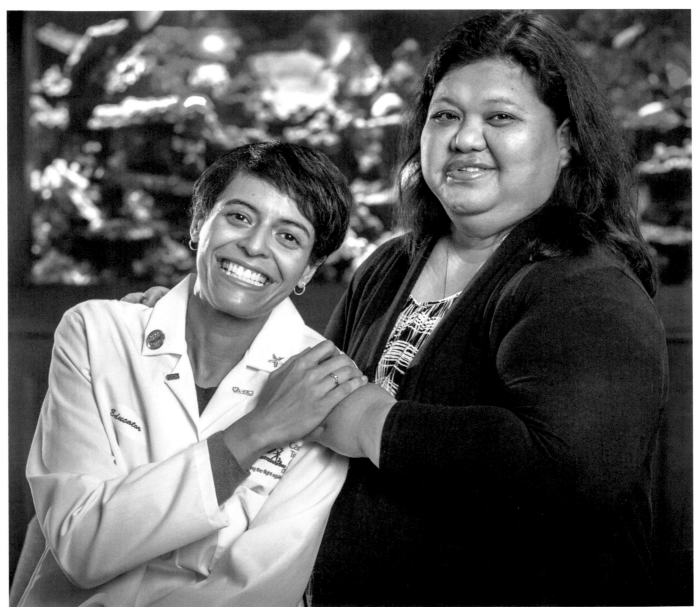

Tahitia Timmons, MSN, RN-BC, OCN, VA-BC, with Juvy Acosta, DNP, RN, ANP-BC [right]

An Understanding Educator

TAHITIA TIMMONS, MSN, RN-BC, OCN, VA-BC [VIRTUA MEMORIAL IN MOUNT HOLLY, NEW JERSEY]

WRITTEN BY JUVY ACOSTA, DNP, RN, ANP-BC

I MET Tahitia in 2009, when she came to work as the staff educator in the medical-surgical oncology unit. We were colleagues and quickly became fast friends. She has a quirky sense of humor and is dedicated to her patients and staff. She is the type of person who cares and puts her heart into everything she does. Nursing was a second career for her. She had started out in sales, but wanted to make a real difference in people's lives.

Peer Tribute

TAHITIA BRINGS a unique perspective to her patients and her staff. After becoming a nurse, she received a diagnosis of a chronic medical condition. This helped give her a patient's point of view. She has experienced some of the procedures her patients encounter. Being a cancer survivor myself, I know that this changes your perspective, and in certain ways, it makes you a better healthcare provider and educator. I believe she has used her experiences in this way.

Tahitia has mentored many of her nurses. She created an orientation program for new nurses that focuses on providing a basic understanding of oncology while also emphasizing the basic skills new RNs need to function effectively in medical-surgery. She doubled the number of chemotherapy/biotherapy nurses and also makes sure the nurses realize the importance of their job.

For Tahitia, this means seeing the patient as a person, not just as a patient. She often says that when she does her rounds, it takes her a long time because she likes to sit and talk with her patients. She told me it's hard to create an equal relationship when you're looking down at someone. She shares this philosophy in her interactions with her nurses. She says that unless you truly care and know something about someone, you cannot teach or empower that person.

She ensures continuity of care by facilitating rounds on the unit and ensuring that the nurses focus on goal-setting. She has worked out a schedule with one of the oncology doctors to present patient case studies so the nurses can have a forum to learn about oncology treatments and diagnoses. Tahitia restarted an oncology nursing practice council to address patient needs. It focuses on quality and encourages the use of evidence-based practices.

Tahitia has touched the lives of many of her patients. For one particular patient, who was going home to receive hospice care, she helped organize a nursing graduation. She worked with the social worker and the woman's school so that, before she died, the woman received an honorary nursing degree.

Another patient had to be hospitalized for a medical event related to radiation scar tissue in the abdomen. Tahitia ensured that she had continuity of care by confirming that her three daughters stayed updated. Two daughters lived in the area, but one lived in the Midwest. The day after surgery, Tahitia facilitated a call with the husband and the daughter in the Midwest, who was also a nurse, so Tahitia could answer their questions.

TEACHING MOMENT:

Tahitia restarted an oncology nursing practice council to address patient needs. It focuses on quality and encourages the use of evidence-based practices.

These are just two examples of so many things she has done for patients. I have known her to bring a patient a favorite sandwich or a special ice cream. When Tahitia injured her heel, one of her patients sent her flowers. She was surprised, but I wasn't. Her patients appreciate her kindness and care. She is always willing to help and always has a kind word (or piece of chocolate). She embodies the spirit of nursing: compassion, caring, quality and a willingness to give your time to help others. As far as cancer nursing, it seems it chose her, and it is a very good fit. ❧

CHAPTER 3
For a Loved
One

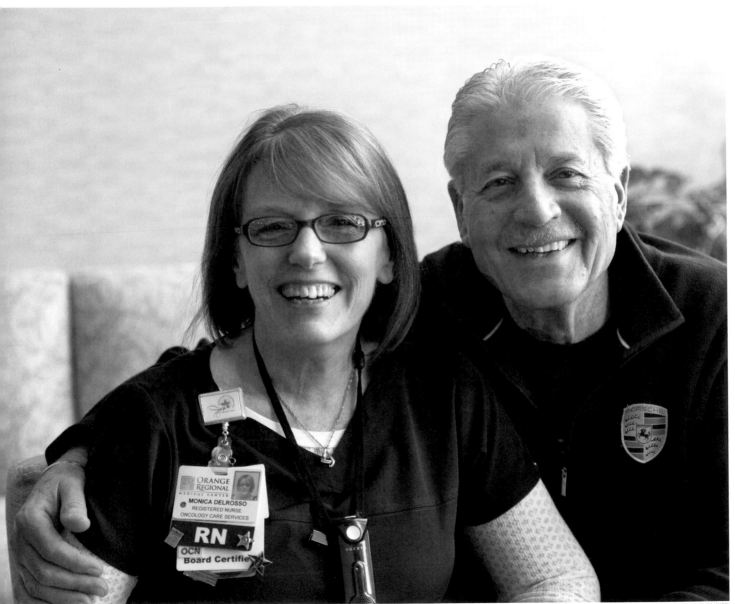

Dan Testa and Monica Del Rosso, RN, BSN, OCN

Generous Care, Generous Gift

MONICA DEL ROSSO, RN, BSN, OCN [ORANGE REGIONAL MEDICAL CENTER IN MIDDLETOWN, NEW YORK]

WRITTEN BY DAN TESTA

I FIRST MET Monica Del Rosso in early September 2011. My brother Larry had just undergone cancer surgery on his left lung, his second operation in three months.

MONICA WAS Larry's nurse his first day in the oncology ward. As soon as I met her, I knew there was something special about her. She knew Larry's history of two operations in three months, so her attentiveness to his needs was outstanding. I have never met a more caring, dedicated nurse than Monica. What impressed me even more was that she would arrive early to discuss Larry's status and leave late to make sure that the new duty nurse was aware of any changes in his condition.

Larry was admitted to the hospital two additional times after his operation, in September and again in late November. During both stays, Monica remained true to form, going way beyond the call of duty. Not only was she caring and accommodating to Larry, she also treated our family and friends with the highest level of comfort and support.

Larry's final visit to Orange Regional Medical Center was on December 14. At the time, we didn't realize it would be his last. Over the next six weeks, until my brother's passing on January 26, Monica was an angel. The level of care she provided Larry and the support she gave us during this difficult time was extraordinary.

Larry's final day was extremely difficult. Monica had arrived early for her 7 a.m. to 7 p.m. shift. She knew his time was limited, so she spent most of her day with Larry, while providing comfort, love and support to our family. At 7 p.m., she remained with Larry and our family until he passed, at 9 p.m. But Monica's day wasn't over yet. She comforted us until we departed at 10 p.m., and then waited an additional hour for the funeral home to take Larry, as we requested. After that, Monica had to complete her paperwork before leaving the hospital around 1 a.m., knowing full well that her new day would start in six hours. You just don't find

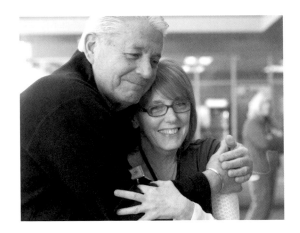

people that caring and considerate. Clearly, it was an extraordinary act of kindness and love.

Monica and our family have stayed connected, and we feel blessed that she remains part of our lives. Larry truly loved her, so he did something very special. Larry donated $1 million to the Orange Regional Medical Center Foundation. In a letter to the president of the foundation, he wrote about the special care he was receiving from the entire nursing staff, especially Monica, and the extraordinary care and support she provided to all of us. ❧

TEACHING MOMENT:

I have never met a more caring, dedicated nurse than Monica. What impressed me even more was that she would arrive early to discuss Larry's status and leave late to make sure that the new duty nurse was aware of any changes in his condition.

Extraordinary Ellen

ELLEN BERG, RN, MSN, OCN [RUSH-COPLEY CANCER CARE CENTER IN AURORA, ILLINOIS]

WRITTEN BY CINDY BANCROFT

I FIRST MET Ellen Berg when we were volunteering for the same program at our children's school. We had the opportunity to get to know each other and to talk casually about her profession. In those conversations, I saw the level of commitment and dedication she has for her patients. I never thought anyone from my family might become one.

MY HUSBAND, Mark, received a diagnosis of Hodgkin lymphoma in early 2008. After he underwent chemotherapy, I cried tears of joy when I learned that Ellen would be the radiation oncology nurse working with us for the next part of our journey. Ellen embraced us and took the time to teach us. She prepared us for the radiation and what to expect. She was that smiling, friendly face we regularly saw when we went day after day for his treatment.

When, a few months later, Mark showed signs of cancer recurrence, I reached out to Ellen, and again, she was right there for us. She helped arrange to get us in with a spectacular doctor the next day and had Dr. Kaushik Patel reviewing Mark's medical records the day I called her. Again, she was always supportive, empathetic, friendly, compassionate and genuine. Every patient can tell when a caregiver is genuine, and that is the most accurate way to describe Ellen.

I clearly remember an early conversation I had with Ellen, when she told me that when she gets cancer, she will have Dr. Patel for her doctor. I was stunned and asked why she would ever say "When I get cancer." She told me that she is no different from her patients and that she sees good, strong, faith-filled people every

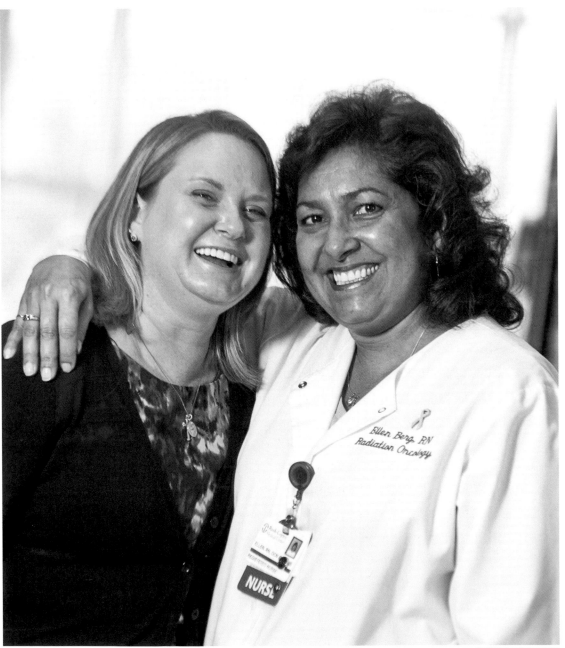

Cindy Bancroft with Ellen Berg, RN, MSN, OCN

day deal with this disease. Why should she be any different than they are? That is Ellen. She is so humble and gracious, and she embraces us as though we are family. Ellen never avoids the difficult conversations. And she always makes the time to be sure that you leave those difficult conversations with a full understanding of the situation and a clear feeling that you will never be alone on this journey.

Once Mark's lymphoma recurred, there was no more radiation in his treatment plan, but Ellen stayed in touch. She always greeted us when we saw her, and I know she was part of our "CarePages" family. When I saw her in church, our eyes would meet, and I knew she was praying for us and our family.

It was a sad day, not even a year later, when I heard that Ellen's oldest son had developed cancer. I found myself remembering our conversation about how her patients are just everyday people and there was no reason to believe that any family would be immune to a brush with cancer. Still, I felt certain she never thought it would be one of her boys. My admiration has grown for Ellen as I have watched her care for, advocate for, and nurse her son. When I see her, I see the same eyes that already had so much compassion and caring for the people who deal with this disease, and now there is even more clarity, strength and understanding behind them. She has set a beautiful example of dignity for all of us.

Anyone who knows a nurse personally knows that this is a profession where the best of the best are dedicated to the care of others. When it comes to oncology nurses, the bar is raised higher.

If I were to describe Ellen Berg, I would use terms like caring, motivating, compassionate, knowledgeable, empathic, embracing and dedicated. If I were to describe what she did for us, I would tell you she made us feel informed, cared for, connected, strong and hopeful. She helped us tell our children what to expect. What more could anyone possibly ask for in a nurse?

My husband and I have said many times that we do not know why he was chosen to take this journey. We also both acknowledge that there have been good things that we may never have noticed in our lives, had it not been for his illness. Ellen Berg is definitely one of those good things. ❧

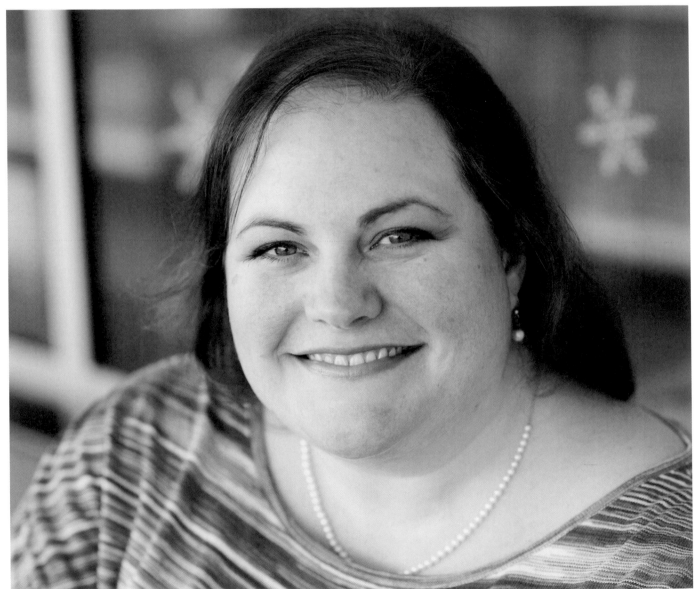

Michelle Knowles, APRN-BC

Someone to Lean On

MICHELLE KNOWLES, APRN-BC [TUCKER GOSNELL CENTER FOR GASTROINTESTINAL CANCERS AT MASSACHUSETTS GENERAL HOSPITAL IN BOSTON]   WRITTEN BY DIANE LEVINE, RN, MPH, CHES, CCRP

FOR SEVERAL MONTHS now, I've been holding on to one of those generic follow-up patient satisfaction surveys from Mass General Hospital in Boston, intending to write something nice about Michelle Knowles. I'd found the survey in a stack of mail that had been sent to my brother, Rick Hagey, who passed away of liver cancer at a hospital in New York City on August 31 last year. Before I could ever get around to that, I ran across the Extraordinary Healer Award in an issue of *CURE*.

For a
Loved One

I FEEL THAT nominating Michelle is befitting not only because of her level of professionalism, but, most importantly, because of her humanity. Michelle Knowles is an oncology nurse practitioner for Dr. Andrew Zhu at Mass General. I have never met her face-to-face, but I can tell you that she is a remarkable and truly compassionate nurse, who goes far above and beyond the basic, mandatory duties of her job. I am a nurse myself. I would know.

To appreciate my story of how exceptional Michelle is, you first must understand a little about my beloved little brother, Rick, who died too young, at the age of 49. It would be difficult, but if I had to sum up my brother in just a few words, they would be: complex, scary-smart, a graduate of the University of Chicago and MIT, talented, witty, intellectually curious, handsome, a critical thinker, well traveled. Rick's demeanor could come off as a bit harsh at times, but deep down he was sensitive and caring. In other words, Rick wasn't someone who was easily won over. You had to earn his trust, especially regarding his personal health care.

Michelle had earned Rick's trust. He told me so. Last year, Rick was living in Boston and commuting to New York City from Monday through Thursday to work. He had never been married, had no children and wasn't currently in a relationship. He'd finally come to the realization early in the summer that his cancer had spread outside his liver and that he might not live another year. He made the difficult decision to come home to Nashville and live with me and my husband to be near our mother, other family members and friends. I was his only sibling.

It took us months to work out the timing and logistics of this move, which was to occur the weekend before Labor Day. Rick and I communicated frequently by phone and email during the summer. It was a most difficult time for both of us. Rick suffered the physical and emotional pain of his cancer alone for the most part, since I was the long-distance caregiver and could offer only verbal support. Rick began to copy me on email strings between Michelle and him to keep me in the loop as to how he was doing and what he was experiencing.

I observed how promptly Michelle would reply to him and that she would often respond outside normal business hours, such as late in the evenings and on weekends. Her tone was helpful and comforting in an

TEACHING MOMENT:

I observed how promptly Michelle would reply to him and that she would often respond outside normal business hours, such as late in the evenings and on weekends. Her tone was helpful and comforting in an honest and sincere manner.

honest and sincere manner. On Thursday, August 23, Rick checked out of his hotel in New York City and made it to the building where he was working. He collapsed in the lobby and was taken by ambulance to a local hospital, where he died a week later.

I went to New York the following day, once the severity of Rick's condition was made known to me. Although we all knew that my brother had a terminal illness, it was nevertheless shocking and devastating that his condition would deteriorate so suddenly and drastically. I immediately reached out to Michelle by phone, seeking clarity, advice and consolation. As it turned out, Michelle was off work that final week of Rick's life, yet I was always able to contact her by phone. In fact, she even gave me her personal cellphone number and encouraged me to call her at any time.

I don't recall her ever saying whether she was on vacation or on leave for personal or family reasons, but she took a good bit of her time off to help and console me during that most awful of weeks. We spoke by phone on several occasions, and her calmness and thoughtful deliberation lent much clarity to the choices I was being asked to make as Rick's healthcare proxy. I can never thank her enough for keeping me from totally coming apart during that period.

My brother never made it to "the finish line," as he referred to getting back to Nashville. He died in an unfamiliar hospital in New York City, on the last day of the lease on his Boston apartment and one day before my husband and I were to bring him back to Tennessee. Rick had a painful, stressful, terrifying and lonely cancer journey, but Michelle was there when family couldn't be, going the extra mile to leave needed prescriptions where Rick, who had an insane travel schedule, could pick them up after hours, and offering advice and consolation. Michelle's special attributes of patience and true compassion serve to help keep me cognizant and mindful that every single patient and visitor I see walking the corridors of Vanderbilt University Medical Center, where I work as a research nurse, could be experiencing as much pain and trauma as I did while tending my brother in New York City. I hope that someday I have the opportunity to meet Michelle face-to-face and give her a huge hug of appreciation for all that she did for Rick and for me. ❧

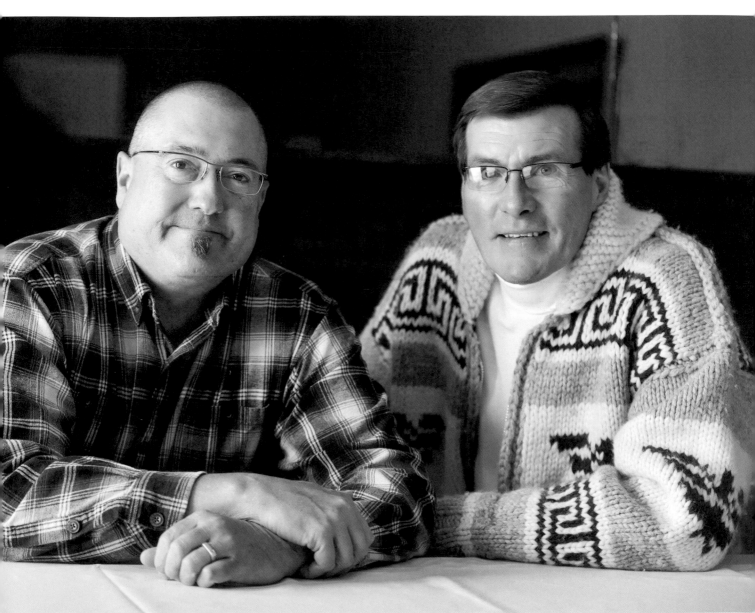

Patrick Silovich, RN, BSN, with David Seeler [left]

Nurse, Neighbor, Friend

PATRICK SILOVICH, RN, BSN [MASONIC CANCER CENTER AT THE UNIVERSITY OF MINNESOTA IN MINNEAPOLIS]

WRITTEN BY DAVID SEELER

MY WIFE, Betsy, received a diagnosis of stage 4B lymphoma in November 2012, after months of misdiagnoses. Several doctors believed that she was having gastro-intestinal problems, but they never did an abdominal scan. Eventually, this test was completed, and the tumors were immediately evident.

For a
Loved One

BETSY HAD stage 1 lymphoma more than seven years earlier that had been treated with surgery and radiation. Her current type can only be treated with chemotherapy. She was very ill due to the pressure that the abdominal tumors were placing on her small intestine and because of chronic anemia. She was scheduled to receive six rounds of a chemotherapy cocktail, one every three weeks. After the first round, her doctor added a biologic agent to the regimen, which is when Patrick Silovich comes into the picture.

Patrick is an oncology nurse who works in the infusion center at Masonic Cancer Center. He has been an oncology nurse for more than two decades. He started out in the Air Force and then became a civilian air traf-fic controller. When that job ended, in the 1980s, he decided to go into nursing. He told us that he had planned to do that for only a few years and then become involved in the pharmaceuticals business. He loved oncology nursing so much that he never left it. He started working in North Dakota and then moved to Minnesota and the University of Minnesota. The first time we met Pat, his confident presence helped to ease the concerns that Betsy and I had. The prognosis for her type of B-cell lymphoma with Hodgkin was not that great. It was the day that the biologic agent would be added to her chemo regimen, and she was especially apprehensive.

Betsy was still very ill, and she felt that the first round of chemo had just about killed her. Adding another drug that would extend her already-long chemo day by two hours did not seem appealing. But Pat had seen that Betsy's first round of chemotherapy had caused some significant tumor lysis and he continued to be upbeat. Pat has a very friendly, confident manner, and it turns out that he and his wife live in the same small community, Forest Lake, as Betsy and me.

Pat explained the drug to us completely and asked if we had any questions. We were concerned because Pat had told us that a percentage of people have a reaction to it. He assured us that he would be ready to do what was necessary if that should happen. On the infusion pump pole, he hung a small plastic bag containing drugs, including a steroid that he would use if Betsy had a reaction. Well, she did have a reaction. Her face started to tingle, and her mouth and lips felt funny. She called for Pat, who was there in a second, shutting off the biologic agent and administering the drugs in the little plastic bag. In less than 15 minutes, Betsy was fine. Pat explained what had happened and that he would start the drug again after about 20 minutes but at a much slower rate. He said some people react twice, which is what happened, but he was right there ready to fix the problem when it did.

TEACHING MOMENT:

Pat is a cheerleader for his patients. And I do mean "his" patients.

Since our first meeting, Pat has been a great supporter with his confidence, humor and compassion. He has made the extra effort to be Betsy's oncology infusion nurse for each of her cycles, which has meant a lot to us. Pat is a cheerleader for his patients. And I do mean "his" patients. He takes direct responsibility for their care the entire time that he is with them. Pat has called our home several times to make sure that follow-up appointments after each cycle were set up and that they were at the correct times.

Betsy has her sixth chemo session this Friday. Her scan shows "no metabolic activity" in the many tumors that she had. At her last chemo session, Pat said, "I hope that I get to be there at the graduation," meaning the final scheduled chemo. Pat has made an amazing difference in our experience, which at first was full of anxiety, dread and fear. He helped us endure the ups and downs of chemotherapy with his professional knowledge, expertise and personal commitment to his patients. ❧

Kenny's Girlfriend

BLANCA VARGAS, RN, BSN, OCN [CRETICOS CANCER CENTER AT ADVOCATE ILLINOIS MASONIC MEDICAL CENTER IN CHICAGO]   WRITTEN BY RON STEMPKOWSKI

NURSES ARE HEROES. There is no doubt in my mind. Nurses who devote themselves to caring for people who are battling cancer are a special kind of hero— an elite force who lovingly carry out their duties regardless of how the mission might end. Their dedication is as unyielding as it is impressive.

BLANCA VARGAS is a first-class example of this type of hero. Her presence at the Creticos Cancer Center transformed the infusion room from a cold, sterile facility into a place filled with caring and laughter—and even a touch of coziness.

For my husband, Kenny Anderson, Blanca was the face of his infusion treatments at Creticos. Her reassuring smile. Her cooing voice. Her gentle yet capable touch. He never looked forward to the treatment, but always looked forward to seeing "his" Blanca. Her warmth drew us both in and earned her a place on the highest shelf in our esteem.

I accompanied Kenny to most of his treatments during the year he underwent them. I can still remember meeting Blanca for the first time, as she prepared Kenny for his first chemotherapy session. She was so sweet and jovial as she donned the required and intimidating hazardous materials garb. She made the whole daunting process seem a little more routine, easing the minds of two very unnerved gentlemen. It was late winter, and she talked about the promise of spring. It so perfectly demonstrated her optimistic point of view.

Kenny was ever the performer and having a loyal audience helped him pass the time while receiving treatment. Blanca engaged him in conversation, listened intently as he shared stories, and she shared stories of her own. It wasn't long before Kenny and Blanca became the best of "dancing" partners as they played off

For a
Loved One

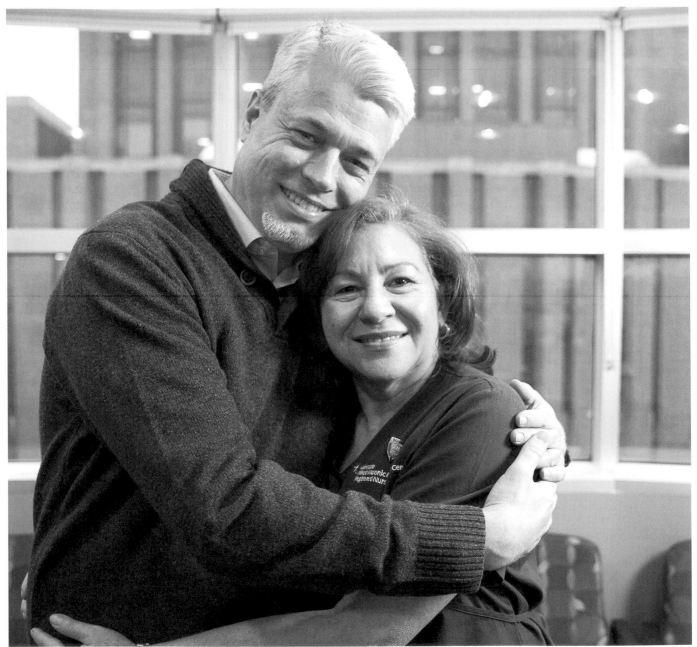

Blanca Vargas, RN, BSN, OCN, with Ron Stempkowski

each other effortlessly, usually resulting in uproarious laughter from their adoring audience—among which I was lucky to be a part.

Their mutual "crush" soon became so obvious to me that I began referring to Blanca as Kenny's girlfriend. And not long after, she and the entire staff were in on the secret. Their affinity for each other was palpable—and so delightfully palatable. No matter how poorly he was feeling as I drove him to treatment, I always loved to watch his demeanor transform and lighten when he saw Blanca. It was a delicious treat for me and one that was so good for him.

With Kenny (as with all her patients, no doubt), Blanca understood the subtle yet powerful importance of touch. I can still see the serene smile that brightened his face when she touched his arm or gently rubbed his back, murmuring sweet words of encouragement.

As Kenny's husband and partner, I watched, helplessly, as either cancer or chemotherapy devastated his body. I was his constant—albeit stressed out—caregiver, and taking him to the treatment center was a respite for me, knowing that Blanca would tend to his every need and give him every indulgence. She understood not only what Kenny was going through, but what I was going through as well. I could breathe a little easier while we were there.

As Kenny's condition deteriorated, he remained steadfast in his optimism—as did Blanca. I so

TEACHING MOMENT:

No matter how poorly he was feeling as I drove him to treatment, I always loved to watch his demeanor transform and lighten when he saw Blanca. It was a delicious treat for me and one that was so good for him.

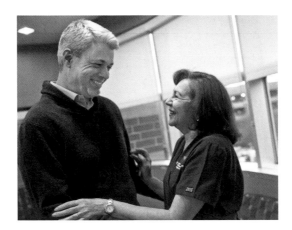

appreciated having another pylon to stand strong with me in support of Kenny. We knew we were going to lose him, but focusing on it would have been paralyzing to him, me and our family. She was such a great help to me in that regard. Knowing she'd cared for so many patients who had ultimately died and yet remained so hopeful and positive and light shored up my courage to do the same.

When he was hospitalized across the street from Creticos, Blanca and the other nurses came to visit him. Though his diagnosis of terminal cancer was difficult for us to grasp, Blanca's demeanor didn't change. She was the same, unwavering fan of Kenny that she'd always been. It's that kind of loving consistency that I found remarkable. Yet she is but one star among a constellation of other professionals who together spun a lattice of care around my Kenny as he valiantly battled cancer.

Since Kenny died, I still visit my heroes at Creticos at least twice a year, taking them the same home-baked goods I brought when Kenny was undergoing treatment. As soon as anyone on the nursing staff sees me, their face brightens and they squeal, "Blanca will be so happy to see you!" before going off to find her for me.

Though the first couple of times were bittersweet—the wounds from losing Kenny were fresh—Blanca is the kind of person you just can't help hugging. Now, it's like going to see an old friend. And that's exactly what she is.

Except my friend is also my hero. ❧

CHAPTER 4
Life & Laughter

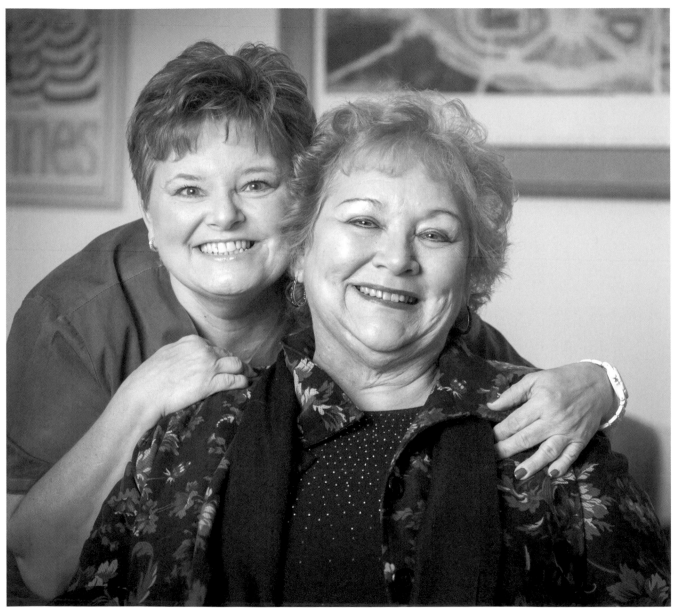

Susan Deeney, RN, BSN, OCN, with Sandra M. Haines [right]

Healing With Laughter

SUSAN DEENEY, RN, BSN, OCN [BURLINGTON COUNTY HEMATOLOGY ONCOLOGY IN WESTAMPTON, NEW JERSEY]   WRITTEN BY SANDRA M. HAINES

AS I ARRIVED FOR my first chemotherapy appointment, my teeth were chattering, my palms were sweating and my stomach was churning. An angel of a nurse named Susan Deeney introduced herself and asked me if I was nervous. After I nodded my head, she told me that if she was having chemotherapy, she would be nervous, too. She explained it was a normal reaction. She offered me something to ease my anxiety and explained she would administer it during my treatment. It was an offer I couldn't refuse.

SUSAN STARTED the treatment, explaining every drug's name, its effects and the time it would take to administer it. She suggested I bring a family member with me during treatments. I explained that my husband was a 100 percent disabled Marine. My other family members were very busy, and I would not impose on them.

Reporting one day for treatment, I was stressed out. Susan asked what was happening. I told her that I'd noticed how busy all the nurses were, but I didn't want to be late for work after chemotherapy. She apologized on behalf of the nurses and offered to come in early for my future treatments.

Another time, I complained about all the things I could be doing while getting chemotherapy. She suggested I use the time to make "to do" lists, clip coupons, watch a movie or read a good book.

One day I arrived a little late for treatment because my husband had had a bad morning. Susan sat down next to me and listened as I told her my problems. Every time after that, she would ask how my husband was doing. When I complained that without my hair, I looked like a Holocaust victim, she said this was my opportunity to have any color hair I wanted. With a wig I could be a beautiful blonde or a flaming redhead or a smart brunette.

Every time I came to the oncology center, Susan would be telling funny stories about her life, like the time she had a personal trainer. (She was prepping for a marathon for a special cause.) Often she would complain that he was working her too hard. One day, while she was working out with the trainer, they saw a group of Marines, who looked exhausted, in a nearby park. Her trainer told her to run fast in front of the Marines; it was her "time to shine." After all, she could show them how to do it. She obliged, and the Marines were stunned to see a middle-aged Susan running past them. We all laughed at her story.

Another day we heard the story about the time Susan and her daughter went to a spa together and came out with face masks and their hands covered with large mittens. Both daughter and mother couldn't stop laughing at each other. All the patients enjoyed her wonderful stories. We all looked forward to them as she took the "ouch out of grouch."

I told her that she was "special" to handle cancer patients on a daily basis and that I couldn't do that type of work. She said she thought I was "extra special" to be a caregiver for a disabled husband on a daily basis and work a full-time job.

It was Susan who would go out of her way to greet me, ask how I was doing and listen to what I had to say. She was instrumental in the care of cancer patients. She would offer to bring us coffee and treats during chemotherapy. Nothing was too much for her. Her personal stories and laughter cheered us all up.

On my last day of chemotherapy, my chemo chair had a congratulations sign on it. Everyone on staff signed it. Of course it was Susan's idea to decorate and acknowledge my last treatment. She always made me feel like a major part of the team.

Looking back, Susan made me aware of how life is to be cherished and good memories are to be shared. Leaving the oncology center, I knew I was losing my safety net, but I had gained a friend. ❧

My Florence Nightingale

VANNA DEST, MSN, APRN, BC, AOCN [HOSPITAL OF SAINT RAPHAEL IN NEW HAVEN, CONNECTICUT]   WRITTEN BY NICK SULLO

HERE I WAS at the top of my career, breezing through life and BANG—I received a diagnosis of stage 4 non-Hodgkin lymphoma. I was stopped in my tracks. I was told I needed to receive chemotherapy at our local hospital as soon as possible.

IN MY FIRST encounter at Hospital of Saint Raphael in New Haven, Connecticut, I was greeted by an oncology nurse—a smiling Vanna Dest. She explained to me the treatment process I was to undergo and walked me through the issues with the chemotherapy and how I could best get through them. She administered the drugs with compassion; she would hold my hand when I was nauseous and always encouraged me to get through this horrendous and physically debilitating treatment.

The chemo caused me to experience severe vomiting and weakness as well as many other struggles. The fear of survival was smacking me in the face. But the process would have been much more difficult without Vanna. She not only administered my chemo but also conferred with my oncology physician throughout my treatment to examine ways to keep me as comfortable as possible. She even came up with ways to alleviate my stress.

For example, I love walking on the beach, so she would tell me during chemo to imagine the sunset, the sound of the ocean waves and the feeling of sand between my toes. Her approach was to have a positive attitude through the process. She kept the word "hope" in all we did, and giving hope to cancer patients has now become a part of my life. I pay it forward by volunteering at our local hospital to encourage other cancer patients as Vanna did for me. Climbing the ladder of success no longer reflects my goals; now, my goals involve helping others.

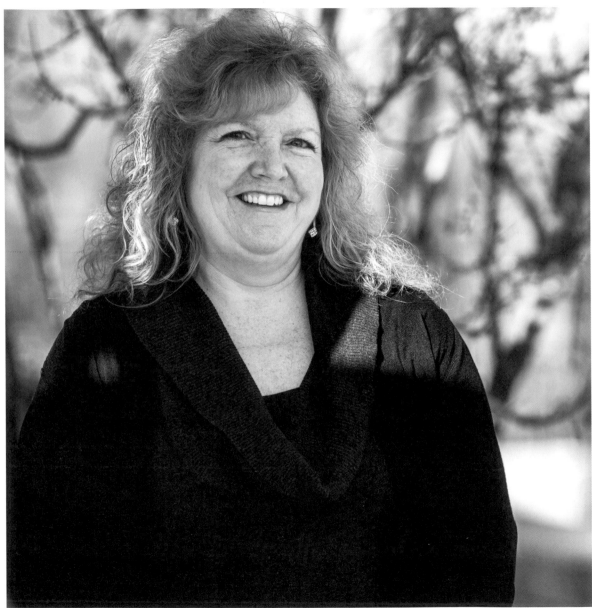

Vanna Dest, MSN, APRN, BC, AOCN

She kept the word "hope" in all we did, and giving hope to cancer patients has now become a part of my life. I pay it forward by volunteering at our local hospital to encourage other cancer patients as Vanna did for me.

Vanna cofacilitated the cancer support group in the hospital. She would give of herself to any and all members. No matter what the issue, Vanna exhibited understanding, patience and awareness of cancer patients beyond the scope of any nursing professional. Her insight into my feelings as I approached the frightening and overwhelming treatment was remarkable. She encouraged me to focus on the positive aspects of this journey, and, believe it or not, there were some positives from having cancer, such as character development and new friendships. She taught me how to strengthen my coping strategies. We attended a laughter seminar for cancer patients because of her. At times, laughter can be our best medicine.

Even after my bone marrow transplantation, Vanna encouraged me to continue my journey through life with hope. I am now cancer-free, but I continue to respect Vanna and her positive inspiration. Vanna continues her journey to help others. After 29 years working at Hospital of Saint Raphael as an oncology nurse and then pursuing her advanced practice nurse certification, she is now working at Smilow Cancer Hospital at Yale-New Haven as the manager of the oncology advanced practice providers and continues to practice as an oncology nurse practitioner. There are many Florence Nightingales out there to help cancer patients; however, I was fortunate to have Vanna as mine. ❧

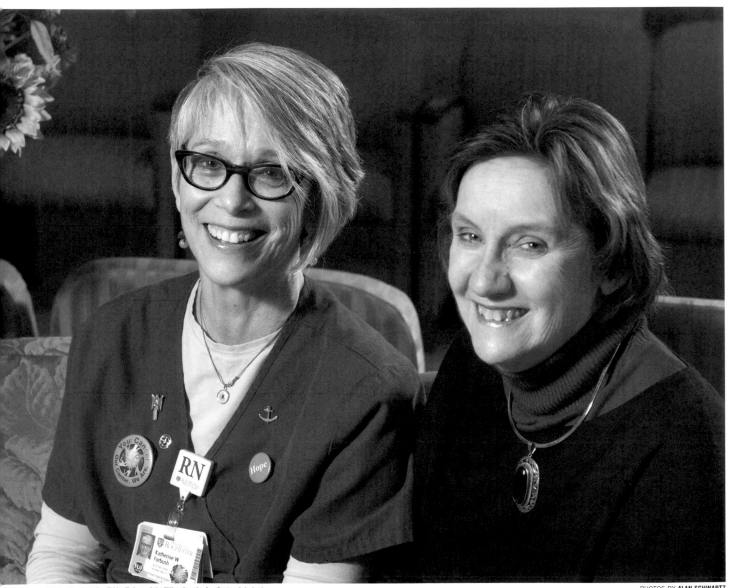

Kitty Forbush, RN, BA, with Elizabeth A. Osta [right]

Team Spirit

KITTY FORBUSH, RN, BA [PLUTA CANCER CENTER IN ROCHESTER, NEW YORK]

WRITTEN BY ELIZABETH A. OSTA

I THOUGHT that the day I was to start chemotherapy for breast cancer would be one of the worst days of my life—instead, it became one of the luckiest.

"THIS IS KITTY," said the head nurse. "She'll be your chemo nurse." I'd chosen to have chemo first to shrink the life-threatening tumor in my right breast. I was shaking and hardly breathing. Putting up a brave front, I followed Kitty to a chair. I kept my eyes averted. There were lots of people in chairs around the room—people getting chemo. I was too scared to look.

"So, what books are you reading?" Kitty asked once I settled in the chair. She wheeled around me on a small stool, bringing trays in place, oozing competence.

"*Name All the Animals*," I said. I saw Kitty's brown eyes widen behind her stylish, black frames.

"The one by Alison Smith?" she asked. I nodded. "That's the story of my life," she said as she pulled her stool in front of me. "My brother died when I was 16. Just like in her book."

I felt my breathing return; my curiosity replacing my fear. I remembered the death that changed Alison Smith's life forever; her parents so lost in grief that they forgot about their daughter.

"My father became an overnight alcoholic. My mother never got over it."

I gasped. Who was this woman who had survived a horrid tragedy and who would be giving me drugs that could kill me?

"I loved that book because it helped me to see my life." She scooted around and, without my realizing it, pulled a metal pole in place, a clear plastic bag hanging from it. "You're having chemo to shrink that darn cancer, right?" I nodded, spellbound. "You've come to the right place."

I smiled. As she positioned the pole and found my recently installed port for the needle, I marveled. Not only was she at work saving my life, but she was also here to save her own. My breathing slowed and deepened. I sat back as she counseled me to stay off the Internet.

"Bring me all your questions. Call me anytime. If I don't know, I'll find out. I promise." She looked into my eyes. "You're a little scared, right?" she asked as she pulled in closer.

I nodded, my eyes filling with tears.

"I get that." She turned to my husband, Dave, who had come in to be with me. "She's doing great. I just told her to call me anytime. You, too, okay? We'll be a team. The three of us."

The room had a dozen chairs, most filled with patients. Kitty looked at me as if I were the only patient in the room. Who is this woman, I asked myself again. How does she do this work?

I found out soon enough. This blonde, 50-something dynamo had been doing this job for 25 years. And loving it.

"It's the patients who keep me sane. You folks are my inspiration," she said one day.

Once cleared for surgery, I had new tests that showed I needed more chemotherapy. I was amazed at the calm I felt. I'd be able to return to Kitty. How did she do it? I was now looking forward to chemo. As she pumped me full of the chemo drug, she sang funny songs, sweet songs and inspiring songs. We caught up on books we were reading. My tears were soaked up in laughter as she scooted around the room, her face full of

TEACHING MOMENT:

My tears were soaked up in laughter as she scooted around the room, her face full of holiday cheer, which brightened the faces of those around her. Hugs in abundance helped ease the heartache of fear and isolation.

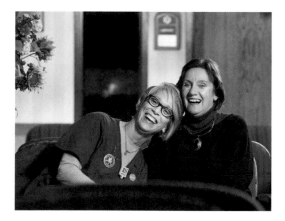

holiday cheer, which brightened the faces of those around her. Hugs in abundance helped ease the heartache of fear and isolation.

When I asked if she thought I would be well enough to be grand marshal at my friend Peggy's ordination in a few weeks, she not only reassured me I could, but when the day came, she surprised me by coming to support me, helping me keep my wig in place.

As my treatments continued, I watched with awe as this petite and vibrant woman wheeled from patient to patient, dealing up deadly drugs with competence and caring. I knew I was one of the lucky ones. The dynamic team of nurses, with Kitty as their comedic star, gave health and humor in abundant doses.

As I pushed through the last of my treatments, I was invited to throw out the first pitch at a Red Wings baseball game for breast cancer awareness. Kitty would sing the national anthem. I did throw the ball, and she filled the stadium with her strong, clear singing. "Awesome," a word she often uses, is one that applies to her.

When I told her of the book I was in the middle of writing when I received my diagnosis, she beamed.

"You'll finish it. I have no doubt."

A year after my treatments ended, I did finish it. It was published the following year.

Kitty sang at the book launch and continues to accompany me to presentations, singing and bringing laughter and love wherever she goes.

A portion of the proceeds from *Jeremiah's Hunger* are donated to Pluta Cancer Center, where Kitty Forbush continues to bring magic and majesty to the healing arts. ❧

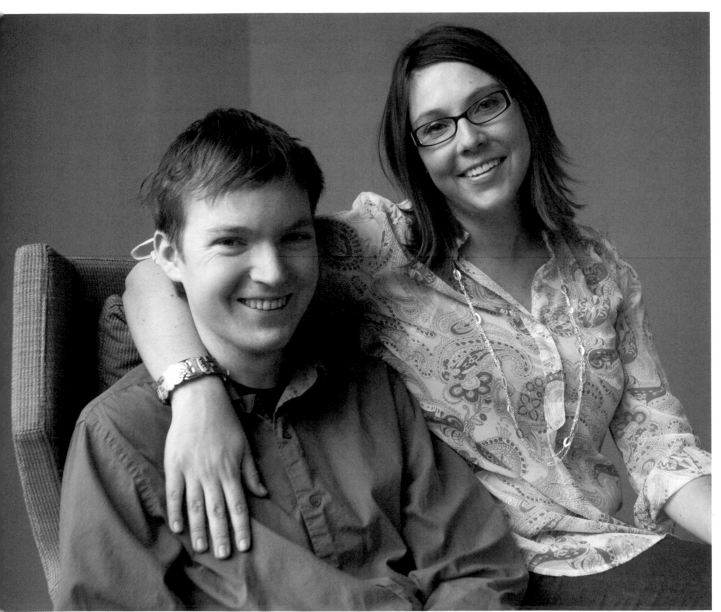

Kyra Erwin, RN, BSN, CPHON, with William Harper [left]

I Had Help

KYRA ERWIN, RN, BSN, CPHON [SEATTLE CHILDREN'S HOSPITAL IN SEATTLE]

WRITTEN BY WILLIAM HARPER

BEFORE JULY 2010, there had never been a reason for me to spend even one night in a hospital bed. But after that summer, the one before what was going to be my last year in college, the Seattle Children's Hospital hematology/oncology unit became my home for the better part of the next two years.

IT WAS TRAUMATIZING, difficult and absolutely terrifying for my family and me to accept the reality of my acute lymphocytic leukemia (ALL) diagnosis. But as unnatural as it felt to be sleeping next to an I.V. pole with beeping chemo pumps, the moments I shared with my weekend overnight nurse Kyra Erwin made a dire situation as close to fun as it could possibly get. She made me laugh every single time she came into my room. And on nights when I was starting a new antibiotic for yet another infection, she would sit on the edge of my bed. When she left, I always knew that things would turn out all right. She supported me when the bad news just kept coming, and she laughed with me whenever we got the chance. When we first met, she was my nurse, but today, she is a dear, dear friend.

Kyra decided to become an oncology nurse after losing her grandmother to breast cancer when she was 14. She told me that "cancer patients just hold a special place in my heart," and that's because she has been touched with the kind of loss that her patients and their families face every day. She gets us, cares for us, has been where we are and always does that little bit more that sometimes makes all the difference.

That place for cancer patients in Kyra's heart must have taken on a whole new meaning after the role she played in fixing mine. She gave me my life when it was so close to being taken away.

When I first got sick, I didn't even know what the word "oncology" meant. I learned fast, though, and

I also learned about other things like infections, neurotoxicity and blood clots. I had those complications and more—so many in fact that even some of my physicians wondered how I was going to get through them. They tell me now that they're impressed by my strength and resilience, and all I can say to that is, "I had help."

On one particular night, less than a month after my stem cell transplantation, Kyra was that help. She alone could tell that there was something very, very wrong with me. My vital signs were normal, but somehow she just knew something wasn't right. When I told her not to leave me alone, she didn't ignore it; I learned later that feeling was what's commonly referred to as "impending doom." When the charge nurse told her not to worry because my vitals were fine, Kyra insisted that the hospital's rapid response team evaluate me. Her relentlessness got me upstairs to the ICU, and not long after that, my blood pressure started to plummet to a low of 50 over 20. I was about to die. An ICU nurse phoned my mother and told her to come in; the nurse didn't tell her why, but when my mother arrived, she saw a medical resident kneeling over me giving me chest compressions. I was about to go into cardiac arrest. The team members stabilized me, and shortly thereafter, they removed a tennis ball–sized blood clot from my pericardial sac. I would have died that night if I had stayed on the unit, but Kyra listened to her intuition and got me the help I was going to need.

I don't know how Kyra could have predicted that things would get as bad as they did that night. Maybe all she knew was that something wasn't right with me, so she did everything she could to get it fixed. If she hadn't, I don't know how else I would have been able to wake up two days later thinking I had been in a car accident. I don't know how I could have graduated from college in May 2012. And I don't know how I would have been able to take a trip to see my family in France during the summer of 2013.

I do know this, though: There are so many people who fought for me when I couldn't do it myself, but Kyra did it when it was only she who had the intuition to know that I needed her help to get me up to the ICU that night. She was more than my nurse; she was exactly the person, the angel, I needed in that moment if I was to have my 22nd birthday six months later. I have many people to thank for that, but Kyra is special to me, because when my life was on the line, she listened to her own judgment.

Thank you, Kyra. You are, and always will be, an inspiration to me. ❧

The Unstoppable Mary

MARY DIBLEY, RN, HP (ASCP) [JAMES P. WILMOT CANCER CENTER AT THE UNIVERSITY OF ROCHESTER MEDICAL CENTER IN ROCHESTER, NEW YORK]   WRITTEN BY MICHAEL J. JASEK

I HAVE LONG been described as a somewhat surly curmudgeon, a fact that makes this essay all the more remarkable. I write to extol the virtues of one extraordinary oncology nurse, Mary Dibley.

IN JANUARY 2010, I received a diagnosis of multiple myeloma. I was being treated by an oncology group practice with a chemotherapy regimen that left me with the expected negative side effects. During this treatment, my oncologist often conferred with Dr. Michael Becker at the Wilmot Cancer Center regarding the potential benefits of a stem cell transplantation.

My appointment with Dr. Becker in June 2010 began with an introduction to a 4-foot-11-inch bundle of energy identified as the blood and marrow transplantation program nurse coordinator. Since that initial meeting with Mary Dibley, I am unable to think of an extended period of time when we have not communicated regarding some medical issue, real or imagined, for which I "needed" an immediate answer. Mary has been stuck with me for nearly four years and has yet to display any annoyance or impatience with my relatively frequent requests for information or a prescription refill. Because of my unrealistic expectations for a continuous source of information, I have just recently forbidden her from taking any time off unless she provides me with a contact number.

At our initial meeting, she exhibited extreme patience and understanding, explaining the process of an autologous stem cell transplantation. Those of us who have gone through this process know how complicated the procedure can become and find it comforting to have it explained in terms that are readily understandable. She instilled a sense of calm in me that enabled me to better understand what I would be facing.

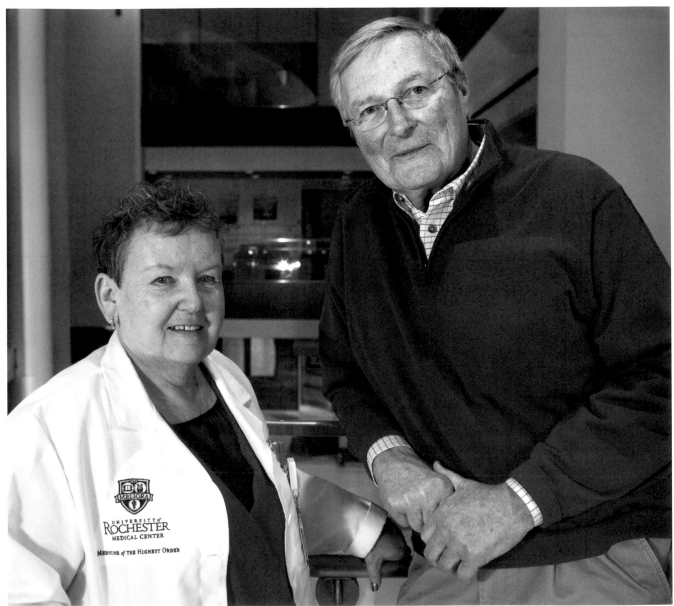

Mary Dibley, RN, HP (ASCP), with Michael J. Jasek

Mary has that rare ability to make you feel as if you are her only patient, when, in fact, hundreds before you have sat in the same room and benefitted from her vast and accurate knowledge. She keeps current by attending seminars and other training opportunities. In fact, her energy in pursuing information concerning recent advances in the fight against multiple myeloma and related diseases is hard to adequately describe.

It is not unusual for me to receive a call from Mary way beyond normal working hours or on weekends in response to a question I've left on her answering device. In addition to her frequently extended stays at work, Mary has filled a most important need for multiple myeloma patients in conjunction with the Rochester Gilda's Club (now Cancer Support Community). Mary donates valuable time to serve as a facilitator for the monthly multiple myeloma support group. She invited me to the support group without fanfare by handing me a card with the date and time of the next meeting. In response to my incredulous look, she said, "I'll see you there next Tuesday." I will never regret my reluctant attendance, as it gave me an opportunity to learn so much from the other participants. The group also instilled in me a much-needed positive attitude I'm sure would be absent without this opportunity. I can't imagine how much information would be missing from our group without Mary's selfless contribution of the time required to keep us up to date with the latest advances and techniques being developed and discussed by health professionals fighting this currently incurable cancer.

Attempting to further describe the wonderful attributes of this vertically challenged nurse (did I mention she does not reach 5 feet?) is way beyond my ability. Sure, I could pore through the thesaurus and find numerous glowing adjectives that would only embarrass this consummate professional. But I would risk sounding too effusive. Just when I thought I knew about most of her volunteer activities, I learned that she had also travelled to the Dominican Republic with a small mission from her church to assist with the review of procedures at a disadvantaged medical facility. Knowledge of all Mary's volunteer activities is not easy to achieve, owing to her self-effacing nature.

If I were forced to describe Mary in one word, it would be "unstoppable." And I do mean unstoppable in every endeavor she has taken on. I could not imagine what my trip through this labyrinth of cancer treatments would be without this loyal and caring human being. ❧

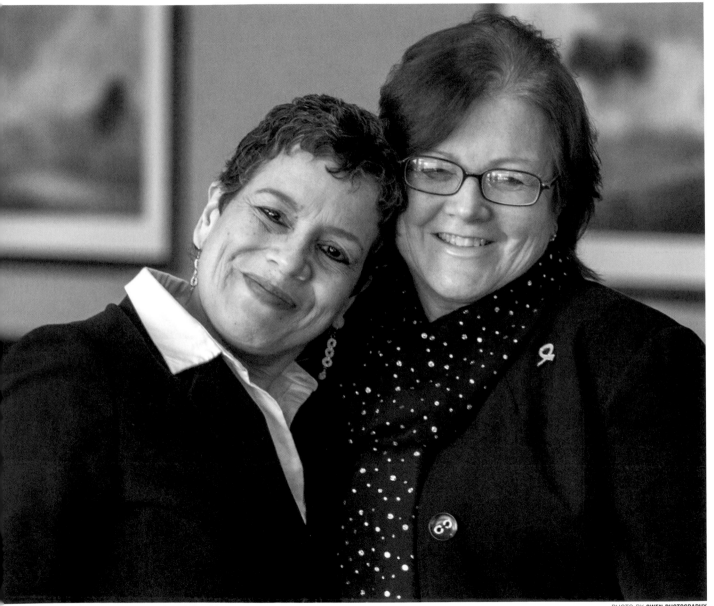

Colleen O'Brien, RN, CBCN, CBPN-IC, with Nancy Gonzalez [left]

My New Breast Friend

COLLEEN O'BRIEN, RN, CBCN, CBPN-IC [WINTHROP-UNIVERSITY HOSPITAL BREAST HEALTH CENTER IN MINEOLA, NEW YORK] WRITTEN BY NANCY GONZALEZ

HEAR YE, hear ye, I have come to sing the praises of nurse Colleen O'Brien!

I HAVE COME to know Colleen through most unfortunate circumstances, unfortunate circumstances that have now awarded me with a new best friend. Or, as we like to say, breast friends!

My name is Nancy Gonzalez. I am 53 years old and have been married for 30 years. I have two grown daughters, ages 20 and 27.

In November 2012, I went for a mammogram that resulted in a biopsy. Consequently, I was informed on December 26, 2012, that I had breast cancer. Needless to say, I was devastated. The day after Christmas? Come on, now!

The hospital called me the next day to ask my permission to forward my name and number to their social worker Michelle DeCastro and their breast nurse navigator Colleen O'Brien. Giving permission was one of the best decisions I ever made.

I was counseled by Michelle. However, I had so many questions regarding the cancer that Michelle would say, "You must speak to Colleen; she will answer all your questions."

So, I called Colleen. I had a list of questions. At that point, I really could not ask too many questions without crying. She was so sweet, compassionate, knowledgeable and eloquent in her explanations. If she was not certain of something, she would say, "Nancy, I will get back to you." And guess what? She did. Almost immediately.

It was about four weeks from the first time I spoke to Colleen to the lumpectomy. She made the most unbearable time bearable. I kept telling myself, and I told her on occasion, God must have sent her to me. How could I have my own personal nurse? I live in New York City! This is unheard of. No one believed me. Oh, I believe. I believe!

The day before the lumpectomy I must have called her two dozen times. I still had not met her face-to-face. But on that last call on Tuesday evening, I started crying and said, "I love you, Colleen. God sent you to help me. I know I'm being a pain, but you have made it so much easier for me."

All my family and friends at work could not believe that I had not met this Colleen about whom I had been bragging, saying, "I love that Colleen."

Finally, the day of surgery, when I was in the recovery room with my eyes closed, I heard someone say, "So, here I am! How are you doing?"

I opened my eyes. "Colleen?"

"Yes," she said.

I said, "You look just like what I'd imagined you'd look like."

"How?" she asked. "An old white woman?" So funny! Just like the woman with whom I had formed that perfect relationship on the phone. She was true to life.

Colleen has been there for me since then, arranging my appointments, educating my husband and me on every step—and there are many—that we have taken. She has been my nurse, sister, best friend, breast friend, mentor and educator on all things breast cancer.

She was there with my husband and me when the oncologist told me I had to have chemo, radiation and take a pill for a number of years. I was totally devastated. I could not believe it. I thought I would just need to have radiation. I sincerely could not comprehend all the doctor was saying. All I could think of was the word "chemo." Dr. Nina asked me, "Nancy, do you understand?" I just turned to Colleen. "Colleen, do you understand? Because I can't understand anything right now. Can you explain it to me later?" She said, "Of course, Nancy." After that we sat together at the pizzeria across the street and had a glass of wine and laughed. Colleen told me, "You can beat this chemo, Nancy."

Not long after, I had my first round of chemotherapy. Colleen was there while I was hooked up. The nurses would come over and say to her, "You know her?" She'd say, "Her? She's my breast friend. Oops, I mean best friend." I have cried to Colleen on the phone so many times I can't count. I never felt embarrassed. She has always been there for me. For all these reasons, she is the best breast nurse navigator in the world. ❧

Hands-On Care

VICKI WILSON, RN [ARIZONA ONCOLOGY ASSOCIATES IN TUCSON, ARIZONA]
WRITTEN BY MAE KRUEGER

"HAVE BREAST CANCER, get free things" is the way I have sometimes described life after a cancer diagnosis. I have received lots of gifts since my initial diagnosis in 2000, including many T-shirts, several sets of pink pom-poms, four months of a cleaning service, a couple of schnauzers, mindfulness and the opportunity to reflect. So I am embarrassed to admit that it wasn't until I saw the Extraordinary Healer Award notice in *CURE* that I recognized one of the greatest gifts breast cancer has brought me—Vicki Wilson, my oncology nurse.

CANCER PATIENTS can be pretty self-focused. We have a lot on our minds. I know, because since 2007 I've been living with breast cancer metastasized to my bones and lungs. (Did you notice how I just cleverly inserted that into this essay, even though it is not supposed to be about me?) But being self-focused has also resulted in taking more time to really notice everything around me and find peace in simple, small things. So, back to this gift in my life—Vicki.

I had the pleasure of meeting Vicki in late November 2000 at my first chemo session. I don't remember the actual meeting, but now that I know Vicki, I am certain it was a pleasure. Part of what is wonderful about Vicki is that she has known me for 12-plus years. With only a few exceptions, she has always personally administered my therapy. As far as I'm concerned, Vicki's mission is to make me believe I am the only patient she actually cares about and for me to never suspect that all the patients around me believe this as well. She

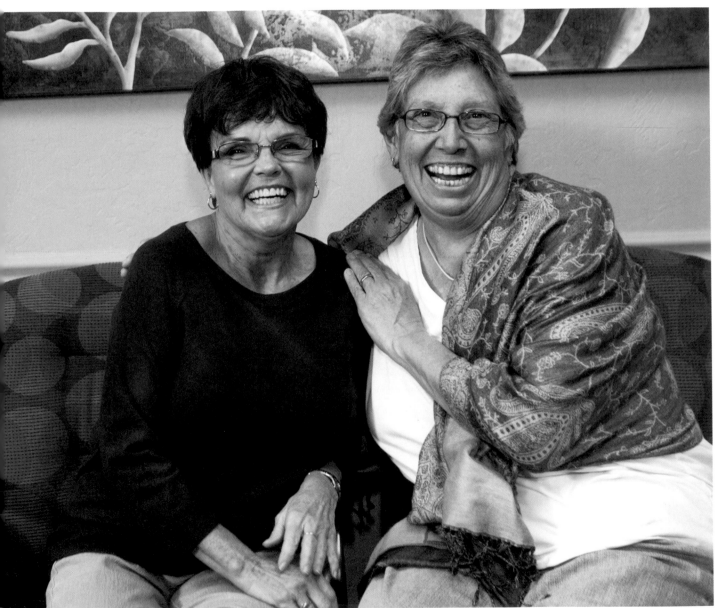

Vicki Wilson, RN, with Mae Krueger [right]

tends not to talk about herself. (And by that I mean that I have been self-absorbed and have never inquired about her life.) Vicki has never felt the need to insert her own experience into the silence following my answer to "Did you do anything fun over the weekend?" Instead, she listens.

So, I admit I don't know if Vicki has ever been married or if she has kids. I don't know if she is a native Tucsonan or a transplant. Here is what I do know. She's speedy. She moves quickly throughout the chemo room, the examining rooms and the office. She is rarely still. She is über-efficient and doesn't miss a thing as she circles and surveys all of us in our chairs. I can hear her taking stock of our progress. "Is that drip finished? Are you cold? Do you need a blanket? Are you still doing okay? You're almost done." It's her domain, her sphere, and she runs the room. She (almost) always has a smile on, and if the smile is missing, it's probably my oncologist's fault. (Sorry, Doc.) She can kid and laugh with the best of them. But her compassion is warm and embracing. She is always kind.

When she comes to me, when it is my turn, I feel as though the sun just poked through the cloud around my head and that everything will be just fine while I'm in her care. I usually end up telling her something that I intended to tell my doctor but forgot. I am more relaxed with her and the length of time I have had her caring for me has made it easy to confide in her.

TEACHING MOMENT:

As far as I'm concerned, Vicki's mission is to make me believe I am the only patient she actually cares about and for me to never suspect that all the patients around me believe this as well.

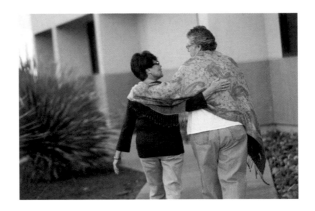

Anyone who takes the time to write about oncology nurses is going to say they are compassionate and kind. Nurses who lack those qualities will simply never be nominated (and probably shouldn't be working in oncology). So, what can I tell you about Vicki that sets her above and apart from other oncology nurses? Her commitment to her work and her efficiency in performing that work make her extraordinary. She makes the best of a bad situation for me and for everyone she tends to. I am listened to, I am heard, I am made comfortable, I am treated quickly but compassionately, and I'm sent on my way with a smile from Vicki that lights up her whole face.

Vicki is starting to think about retirement and has reduced her work hours to three days a week. I "retired" to disability in 2012, so I've been cheering her on. I selfishly want Vicki as the person treating me for the rest of my life. But I want this more: I want Vicki to have time and a chance to reflect, to be mindful and, above all, to have some freedom from work and have a lot of fun.

When I sent the above to Vicki to make sure that she approved of what I had written before I sent it out into the universe, here is what she sent back, which I believe reinforces what I've already told you.

"I guess I have kept a low profile and have never been awarded or sought after any accolades. I have done continuing education and been a member of the Oncology Nursing Society. All I ever wanted to do was direct, hands-on nursing care. Not for me any administrative positions. I tried that early on, and it wasn't for me. I've […] worked oncology for 37 years. Thanks for this, Mae. It means a lot to me." ✤

CHAPTER 5
Touching the Spirit

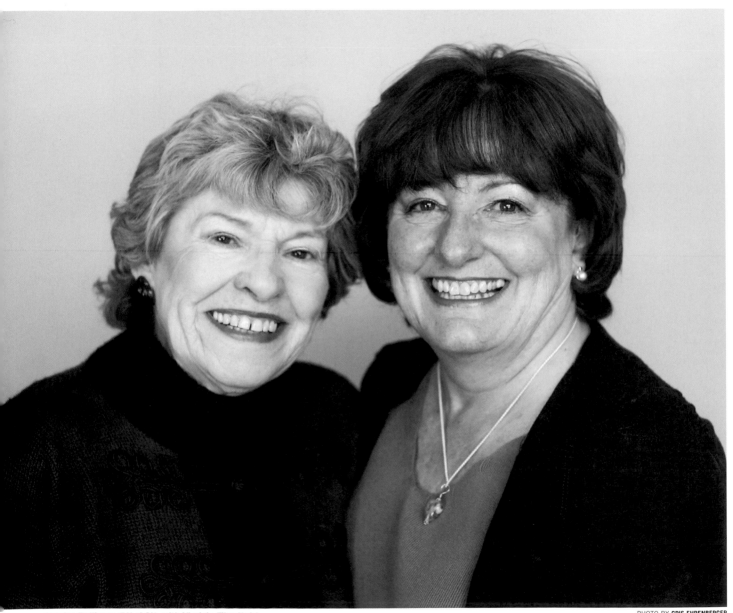

Juanita Bellinger, RN, OCN, with Virginia Filar [left]

The Best Gift

JUANITA BELLINGER, RN, OCN [CANCER CARE ASSOCIATES IN ROYAL OAK, MICHIGAN]
WRITTEN BY VIRGINIA FILAR

IT WAS December 26, and Santa had saved my best gift for last—not under the Christmas tree or in my stocking but at the infusion center. Juanita Bellinger met us at 8 a.m., ready to hold my hand, explain all the procedures, answer any questions and administer my chemo drugs.

I'D ARRIVED fearful and exhausted. It was the day after Christmas, and for two days I'd shared food and gifts with my family as they all said words of encouragement. But none of them had ever experienced chemo in any manner. Admittedly, I was a bit excited to be at a place where my tumors would be attacked and hopefully shrunk, but oh so anxious, not knowing what to expect.

For the next eight hours Juanita was right there—efficient, very attentive and knowing just what to do when the drug caused my body to react adversely. She was calm, comforting, caring and very encouraging for me to go on with the infusion at a slower rate when all signs were in a good range.

For the next three days, I experienced and observed Juanita being the educated, sympathetic oncology nurse to me and all the others there for treatment. When issues arose concerning my mental anxiety or physical comfort, there she was with explanations, reassurance and resolve. She makes sure you have a pillow and blanket if needed and a snack or drink if desired. This experience continued for four days a week every month through June 2009. When it was completed, we parted with hugs, smiles, hope and encouragement.

In May 2010, scans required a return to chemo treatment, due to a rapid growth of tumors. This time it was administered four days a week through October 2010. Cancer Care Associates had closed the office and infusion center 15 minutes from our home and moved to its original main location, a 55-minute drive for us.

Because of the distance, we decided to have three of the infusions at a satellite location close to home. It was new; everyone had a private, quiet, lovely physical space. The staff was made up of good oncology nurses. But there was no warm, fuzzy feeling of deep caring like the one I'd experienced with Juanita.

Until November 2012, my calendar was treatment-free. Then the old two-steps-forward-and-one-step-back reality of cancer reappeared. I was back in chemo. We decided where we'd go because of Juanita. Forget the drive time or cost of gas—Juanita's spirit was worth more than anything else. Because I'd tried different nurses in a different location, I knew there was no substitute for a kind, caring, knowledgeable, smiling, informative oncology nurse like Juanita.

She makes me feel we are part of a strong team. Here we are, four years and three months since we first met, and she is still eager and encouraging about fighting this malady together. Every 21 days, for a series of six treatments, I am greeted by the same dedicated, comforting Juanita, who is ready and waiting to help me and others kick cancer. Because of her, I arrive free of fear and eager to work with the team, knowing she will answer every concern, explain each drug and procedure thoroughly, and patiently search for that one good vein to stick, so we only have to do it once.

But through all this medical stuff, Juanita is such a warm person. We compare gardening advice as well as cooking and shopping tips. She cautions me to watch my diet to avoid nausea and reminds me to drink lots of water to make the pokes successful the first time. She is not only a wonderful, skilled, heartfelt oncology nurse, she is also a good teacher as I know from observing many patients and nurses seek her advice. We are lucky to have her example to learn from and inspire us to carry on.

And so you must agree that on December 26, 2008, I received the gift of an oncology nurse who is truly following her calling. Juanita has lived her vocation by consistently being who she is—a good, professional, caring, competent and up-to-date oncology nurse. In 34 years of nursing, 20 of those as a certified oncology nurse, she has never lost her smile and her generous spirit of caring for each patient as fully as possible. Anyone fighting cancer would agree with me wholeheartedly if only they had the luck of encountering Juanita. ❧

Not Just a Nurse

DAWN MOTES, CMSRN [CRESCENT CITY PHYSICIANS IN METAIRIE, LOUISIANA]

WRITTEN BY CAROL LOPINTO

WHEN WRITING about someone you admire, you instantly think of things to compare them to—guardian angel, hero, lighthouse or calm in the storm. How do you write about the rare individual who is a combination of all these things? She is our soldier, ready to fight at a moment's notice and prepared to fill whatever roles are necessary to make sure we are victors.

I AM A RELIGIOUS PERSON, so when I think of Dawn Motes, I picture a tall, grand, beautiful creature who watches over us. She is adamant about pre-meds and after-meds. She will not compromise anything. She insists on calmness and low stress. She is always watching over her patients and making sure she lessens any side effects. She is prepared for emergencies and knows exactly what to do. She is our guardian angel.

I know everyone has a personal life and would like to leave work and go home to forget about the day, but not our Dawn. She is someone who puts away the self and makes sacrifices for others in their moments of weakness. We are all fighting the toughest battle of our lives, and the uncertainty of the drugs, the side effects and whether we will win this battle makes us feel vulnerable.

She meets with her patients on Day One to make sure they understand everything. She becomes upset if they get nauseated or have pain. She wants her patients to be as comfortable as possible and routinely checks up on them. She gives her cellphone number to call at any time. This is not a service number to page her, but a direct line which she answers with a "Hello, sweetheart."

A few months ago, I was going on a long trip to Missouri with my 16-year-old grandson. I knew I was getting sick the day before, but we had been planning this trip for months; I did not want to disappoint

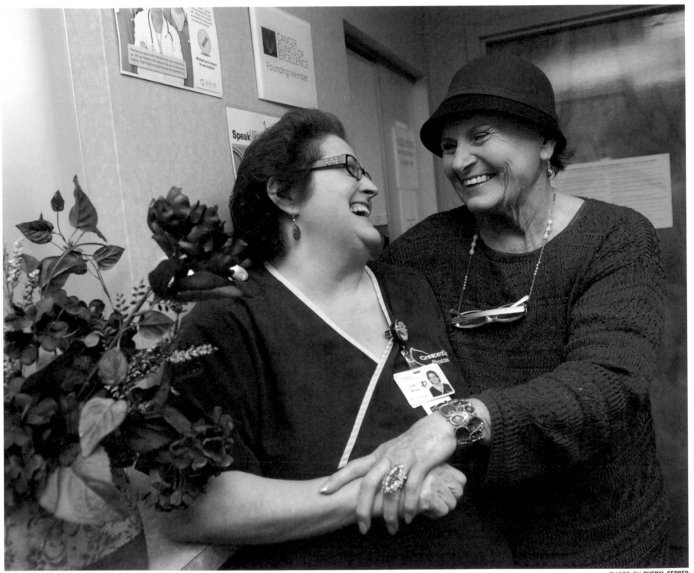

Dawn Motes, CMSRN, with Carol Lopinto [right]

anyone. I do not remember much about that morning, but I am told that I began to become delirious and talk incoherently. When we were about three hours into the trip, my grandson decided to return home. On his way back, he called my daughter, who met us at my home. My temperature was 103.2 Fahrenheit. My daughter called Dawn very early in the morning, before work. Without any hesitation, Dawn told her to give me ibuprofen and proceed to the hospital. The hospital is two hours away. Dawn said to get going and that the emergency department would be waiting for us. Just as she promised, they were.

I can hardly explain how much this meant to us. Our family has been through some extremely rough times in the past two years. First, I was diagnosed with colon cancer two years ago. I was very sick and lost all my hair. I suffered from an *E.coli* infection for many months. I finally recovered, and my hair returned. Then last year, on March 30, my 41-year-old daughter passed away unexpectedly. Just a few weeks later, I was diagnosed with breast cancer. I have had a bilateral mastectomy, and my hair is gone again. That morning when my temperature became dangerously high, my family was very scared and felt unsure how to handle it. Dawn offered a calmness and direction I could never explain. We love her for that.

I know there are many nurses who deserve to be honored, but Dawn is not just a nurse—she is so much more. I have heard patients finishing treatment express their disappointment that they will not get to see Dawn anymore. We love the safe haven she has provided. As our oncologist said, "If you can't get along with Dawn, then you can't get along with anyone." ✤

TEACHING MOMENT:

She gives her cellphone number to call at any time. This is not a service number to page her, but a direct line which she answers with a "Hello, sweetheart."

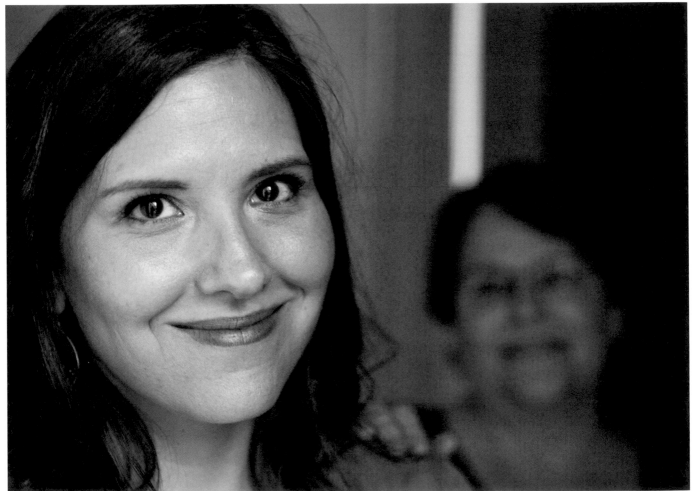

Robin Petro, RN, BSN, with Cindy Kostreba [right]

The Silver Lining

ROBIN PETRO, RN, BSN [COMPREHENSIVE CANCER CENTER AT WAKE FOREST BAPTIST MEDICAL CENTER IN WINSTON-SALEM, NORTH CAROLINA]   WRITTEN BY CINDY KOSTREBA

ON SEPTEMBER 19, 2009, at age 48, I received a diagnosis of stage 3 breast cancer. My treatment included six chemotherapy rounds, a lumpectomy, radiation and a year of more infusions near my hometown, Lexington, South Carolina. After a full year of treatments, I received a diagnosis of "no evidence of disease."

THROUGH INTERNET research and the site ClinicalTrials.gov, I found a trial for a breast cancer vaccine for HER2-positive patients through Brooke Army Medical Center. I immediately contacted the site nearest to me, Wake Forest Comprehensive Cancer Center in Winston-Salem, North Carolina. This was my first contact with my oncology nurse, Robin Petro. Robin was so helpful when I was applying to the trial—answering questions and emails and encouraging me as I anxiously awaited a response as to whether I qualified.

Once I qualified, I met Robin at my first intake meeting at Wake Forest. She had reviewed my huge file and was sensitive to what I had already been through. Unfortunately, I had had a severe I.V. extravasation incident with my port at another facility that had left me with trust issues and white-coat syndrome.

With Robin, I feel as though I really have someone supporting me. She always greets me with a sweet smile and a warm welcome. I look forward to seeing her after my three-and-a-half-hour drive. If she ever has a bad day, which I am sure she does, her patients never know it.

Robin never seems rushed, and on two different occasions when my port was blocked, she was an angel when I became fearful and began to feel faint. Robin responded with cool cloths and calmness, and she brought me back around. Robin didn't make me feel silly, and she was very patient, which helped me to respond well. She always understood my sensitivities with my port. When Robin accesses my veins through my hand or arm, she is so gentle and caring that the experience is painless; it is amazing.

I always look forward to my days at Wake Forest. I have slowly gained back my confidence in the medical community. Words cannot express how much she has helped me handle the emotional and physical side effects of my breast cancer treatments.

My favorite part of the clinical trial was when I came in the first year for injections and the following year for boosters. Those were the days when Robin would sit with me for an hour, taking my vitals and monitoring me for reactions. We would sit and pass the time talking. I began to feel comfortable sharing my experiences, asking questions and talking about my feelings. I shared how I felt when I looked in the mirror and was bald and had gained 25 pounds. I felt I looked so masculine and that I had lost my femininity. These feelings are hard to share with anyone who has not been there, and most medical professionals would not understand. But Robin seems to have an understanding of what her patients are dealing with, which was so comforting for me.

TEACHING MOMENT:

She was an angel when I became fearful and began to feel faint. Robin responded with cool cloths and calmness, and she brought me back around.

Robin also encouraged and supported me when I was preparing to be a speaker at the State University of New York Oneonta's Relay For Life, sharing my experiences and encouraging the college students to support cancer research. Not only do I feel as though I am in control of fighting a cancer recurrence, but I am also actively doing something to help find a cure for others. Robin truly has compassion and understands her patients' physical and emotional health.

Robin is a huge part of the silver lining of my journey. In June 2013, I will have my last booster shot. While I won't miss the long drive each way to Wake Forest, I will most definitely miss my time with Robin. ❧

My New Best Friend

ROBERT H. STEELE, RN, OCN [COMPASS ONCOLOGY IN PORTLAND, OREGON]

WRITTEN BY SHARON STOUT

WHILE I APPRECIATE the kindness and caring of the entire group of hard-working people at Compass Oncology who have taken such good care of me during my cancer diagnosis and treatment, I would like to tell you about one very special individual in particular: Robert Steele, oncology and triage nurse extraordinaire and all-around amazing guy.

THE FIRST DAY I met Robert, I was sitting in the exam room, alone and still a little stunned by the news of my diagnosis. Initially, I was admitted to the hospital on an emergency basis, and after much testing, I was informed I had high blood pressure, anemia, diabetes, blood clots in my lungs—and oh, by the way, "you have cancer."

Dr. Gosewehr came in and made official introductions, telling Robert, "We need to take extra-special care of her." I have no family left, and my best friend of 39 years lives more than 600 miles away, in San Francisco. I thought this was a nice thing for my doctor to say, but I was sure he probably said something similar about all his patients.

I was overwhelmed by the prospect of everything I might need to do to survive, because in addition to a laundry list of other health problems, I had stage 3B ovarian cancer. Of course, I had no idea at that time of all I might need to do, but I did realize I would have to do it on my own. Or so I thought.

Robert handed me his business card and told me he was going to be "my new best friend." I'll never forget it. I didn't know it at the time but have since discovered this to be truer than I could have ever imagined.

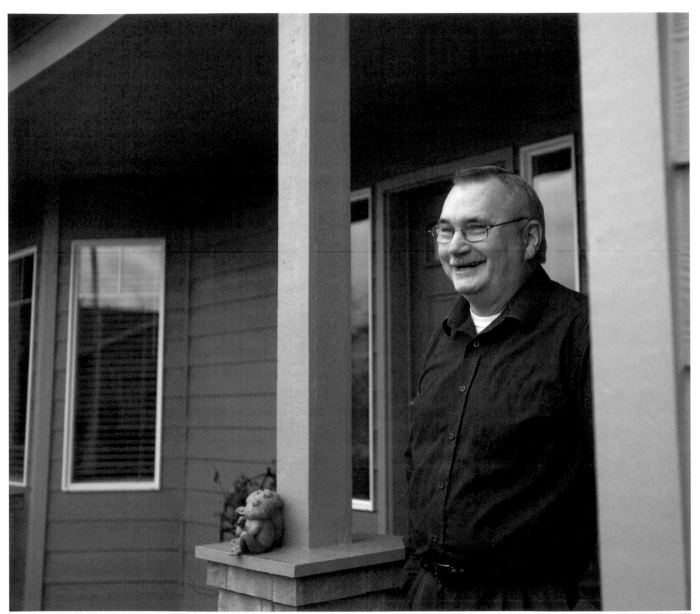

Robert H. Steele, RN, OCN

Robert has taken care of everything and anything I've need as I've gone through 15 months of chemotherapy, surgery and still more chemotherapy. And if that weren't enough, I also suffered a stroke in early January 2010.

I take multiple medications each day, and I can be a little more fuzzy-brained than usual as a result. But because Robert is so good at what he does, he knows what I need better than I do. While I was in the hospital the second time, recuperating from cancer surgery, Robert was on the job. He took care of my every need while I was in a hospital bed and after I had been transferred to a rehabilitation facility.

Robert has helped me with so many things, too many to list here. But in the interest of saving some trees, here are just a few examples: Robert has worked with me, on almost a daily basis, as we tried to tweak the dosage of pain medication I take for peripheral neuropathy. Robert has written letters on my behalf when I missed an important assistance application deadline, and he has helped me apply for financial aid for my many medical bills.

Robert also assists me in the ongoing application process for the drug I take daily. A patient assistance program enables me to receive this medication at no cost, but the program has very exacting application

TEACHING MOMENT:

Sometimes, what I need more than anything is just someone to talk to and to hear me when I'm having a tougher day than usual. I understand how busy he surely must be, taking care of the needs of so many other patients. Robert always makes time for me and has never indicated he's too busy to take care of my latest need or request for assistance.

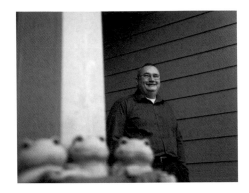

requirements. Robert has taken the time out of his busy day to obtain the application, fill in the appropriate doctor's portion and highlight the patient portion I need to fill in before submitting it for approval within the very specific application window. He even indicates where I need to sign and date it to ensure I submit my part correctly.

Robert does all of this, and more, with professionalism, kindness, compassion and an excellent sense of humor. I often feel bad that Robert seems to be my only source for assistance, again, as my own attempts to assist myself are at times unsuccessful. Sometimes, what I need more than anything is just someone to talk to and to hear me when I'm having a tougher day than usual. I understand how busy he surely must be, taking care of the needs of so many other patients. Robert always makes time for me and has never indicated he's too busy to take care of my latest need or request for assistance. Honestly, I don't know how he does it all.

Even when I thought I had been forgotten by everyone else during this past holiday season, Robert called me on Christmas Eve. He said they were getting ready to close the office early, and he wanted to wish me a merry Christmas. I was so touched that he took the time to think of me and make that call. I don't know if he had any idea I'd be alone, but that gesture meant so much.

I could go on and on about the many things Robert does for me. Suffice it to say that without Robert, I truly don't know what would happen to me. I am currently two years cancer-free, and I'm so grateful to be able to tell the tale. ❧

In It to Win It

LESLEY FERGUSON, RN, OCN   [VIRGINIA ONCOLOGY ASSOCIATES IN NEWPORT NEWS, VIRGINIA]

WRITTEN BY STUART M. EHRLICH

IT WAS early August 2010, during a routine annual physical, when my doctor discovered my hemoglobin level was extremely low. He believed I must be bleeding internally and told me to schedule an upper gastrointestinal endoscopy. The biopsy confirmed an aggressive, malignant stomach cancer. Four days later, doctors removed about two-thirds of my stomach and told me later that the cancer was stage 2 and had spread to the outermost layer of my stomach wall. It wasn't until much later that I fully understood what all of this meant.

AS A 30-YEAR Air Force fighter pilot who must always be ready for combat, I was skilled in the art of survival and trained to endure the punishments of enemy capture, so failure was never an option. At 57, I was in good health and enjoying a good and stable life in the sixth year of my second career, in the defense industry. However, when I was told that I had stomach cancer, I felt hopeless, scared and no longer in control. My loving family—my wife, my three married children and their spouses, and my eight grandchildren—all surrounded me with their love and gave me the purpose and strength that I needed to fight this life-threatening diagnosis. But the uncertainty of the days and months of chemotherapy and radiation therapy ahead of me was uncharted territory, and I was not in the driver's seat—or so I thought.

I first met Lesley Ferguson in October 2010 as I began my six months of chemotherapy and radiation treatments. From our first meeting, Lesley has displayed an active desire to alleviate suffering. Her gift of

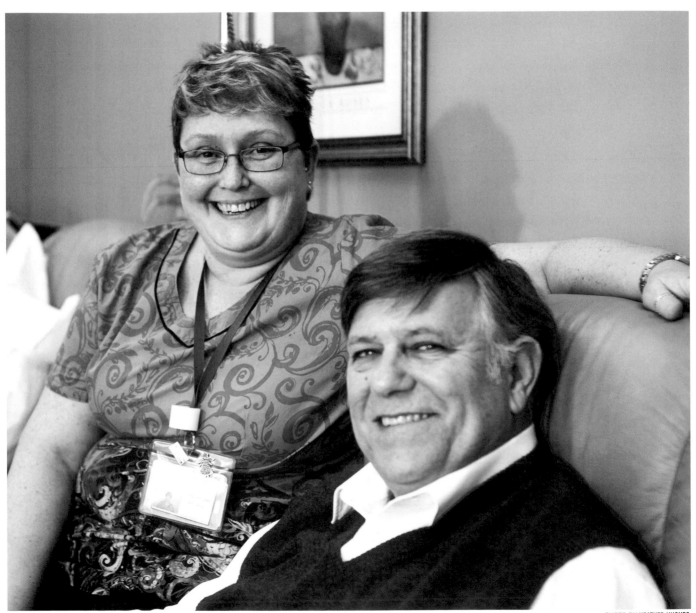

Lesley Ferguson, RN, OCN, with Stuart M. Ehrlich [right]

compassion was unexpected and a comfort to both my wife and me as we began this journey. I wasn't just another patient here to receive treatment; I was here to be cured and to learn from Lesley that it is the quality of one's life that really matters. In a sense, my journey in battling cancer was more of a journey of reflection and discovery about how to live a no-regrets life filled with joy, passion, purpose and fulfillment.

Lesley helped my wife and me prepare for what was going to happen next; she gave us a positive perspective on why we were here. Receiving chemo 24 hours a day, seven days a week, with a tube coming out of my chest, was going to be a big challenge. Lesley patiently answered all our questions and many times anticipated what we might ask and gave us the tools and knowledge we would need.

Yes, I cried when my hair started to fall out and my fingernails began splitting and falling off, but we realized that any remaining cancer cells were also being destroyed—a small price to pay for a cancer-free life. Under Lesley's care there were no surprises; my fear was replaced by peace of mind, renewed hope and a new focus on life.

About six weeks into my treatment, I was feeling unusually tired. Lesley knew exactly what to do. She started me on I.V. fluids before starting my chemo infusion series and told me I could come in any time I needed more fluids in my system. Wow, what a difference that made! I felt so much better.

Her positive and inspiring attitude was contagious not only for my wife and me, but for all the others that she cared for as well. Watching Lesley interact with the other patients was something I wish everyone could see. Perhaps Lesley's greatest qualities are her listening skills and genuine interest in learning who I was as a person. Over the course of my treatment Lesley became much more than my oncology nurse; she became a friend to both my wife and me. She was absolutely the right person at the right time at the right place—she was our beacon of light that guided us through some of our darkest hours, and she smiled joyfully when the doctor told us the great news on July 18, 2011: I was cancer-free.

Lesley is that one in a million who gives so much more than she ever receives. Her warm and reassuring smile, her soft and caring touch, her ability to answer my questions before I even asked, her positive attitude and her enduring and inspiring words "we are in it to win it" have forever been etched into my life. I am a better, stronger and more thankful person today thanks to Lesley! ❧

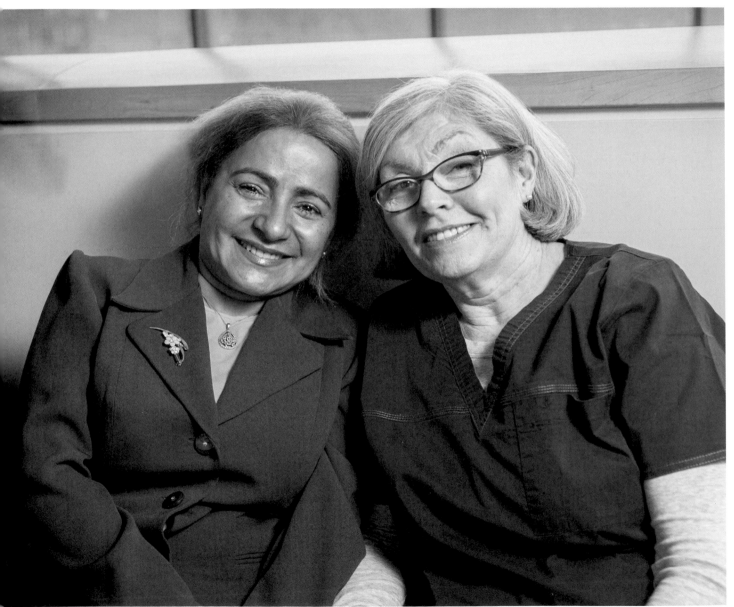

Peggy Guerrera, RN, with Zahra Haghighatjoo [left]

Creator of Love

PEGGY GUERRERA, RN [BOSTON MEDICAL CENTER IN BOSTON]

WRITTEN BY ZAHRA HAGHIGHATJOO

PEGGY GUERRERA is not just great. She is wonderful. What is the best of God's adjectives? How can I explain how much I love her? Without a ceiling, how high is the sky? That is how much I love Peggy.

SHE KNOWS just what I need, at exactly the right time. She knows I love the chemotherapy chair by the sunny window, and so she saves that spot for me. She brings me several warmed blankets and a hot pack for my back before I even ask for it, because she knows I get chilled and have back pain. She knows I need salad because of my special diet and they don't serve it in the chemo clinic. She pays for a salad in the cafeteria herself and brings it for me, not just once, but every time I come in. Even if I am not that hungry, I eat it because I know her extra thoughtfulness in getting it for me. She worries about me all the time. A neck pillow here, cream for my skin, gloves for the cold weather. She anticipates what I need and gives it to me, before I even realize what I need myself.

When I first came to the clinic, I was a Muslim woman from Iran, wearing a scarf. She saw the real person under the scarf. She did not see my color or my religion or the country where I came from. She saw only a person who needed her help and caring touch. She opened up her kind heart to me unconditionally. I am a nurse practitioner in my own country, and I have never known a nurse as kind as Peggy... not even myself!

For every kindness I gave to my patients, my patients prayed for me. I believe their prayers were answered and they brought Peggy into my life. God is creator. Peggy is creator of love. She is a giver. She creates in me compassion and love. Do you want to see God's face on this earth? See Peggy.

There was a very dark time in my life when I honestly didn't feel I could make it another day. At my

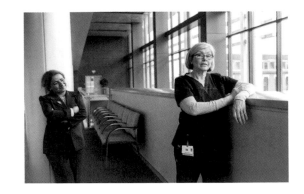

lowest point, I was exhausted and without hope. On that darkest of days, I didn't feel that I could go on. I came to Peggy and explained how I felt, and she wept with me. She and Dr. Hartshorn helped me find the support I needed. Peggy helped me through that day and then called me every day at home to see how I was doing. There is not a nurse in my country who would have done this. Peggy helped me more than you could possibly know.

Everyone at Boston Medical Center, from the door to the top, has treated me with incredible kindness, and I thank them all for that. They are caring and they collaborate with each other. But Peggy is the most special to me. She has helped me to see the importance of humanity and that life is worth fighting for. Every time I come to the clinic, when I see Peggy's face, I see God's face, and I know that I will be okay. ❧

TEACHING MOMENT:

For every kindness I gave to my patients, my patients prayed for me. I believe their prayers were answered and they brought Peggy into my life. God is creator. Peggy is creator of love. She is a giver.

An Unexpected Friendship

NICOLE MESSIER, RN, BSN [VERMONT CANCER CENTER IN BURLINGTON, VERMONT]

WRITTEN BY AMY DEAVITT

ON AUGUST 20, 2003, at 2 p.m., I received the call that changed my life. I heard the words, "We are sorry to let you know, Mrs. Deavitt, you have invasive ductal breast cancer." I dropped the phone and began screaming, "I am dying! I am dying!" My life flashed through my mind. Over and over I saw the faces of my children.

IN THE DISTANCE, I could hear my husband's voice as he spoke to the caller. It took me about an hour to come to my senses and realize that I had just been told me I had a disease that was trying to kill me and that someone would be in touch with a plan. Now, looking back, that was the best thing they could have said. Those words empowered me to take control of the journey on which I was about to embark.

The first call I placed was to the Vermont Cancer Center. I spoke with an amazing scheduler, who tried her best to calm me down, setting my first appointment for 9 o'clock the next morning. It was the longest night of my life.

My angel, Nicole Messier, greeted me after I had checked in. She escorted my husband and me into a small conference room to chat. Her smile was comforting, and her presence commanded my inner calm. I instantly felt her warmth and compassion. She knew we were scared, and she came armed with the answers to the questions we were about to ask.

Nicole had been given advance notice of my condition by my best friend, Kim. Kim was Nicole's day care provider, and she had spent the previous night assuring me that I would be in Nicole's safe hands the next morning. This was one of the many blessings I had been granted over the years.

During the next few days, we spent a lot of time going through all the steps to formulate a plan to take

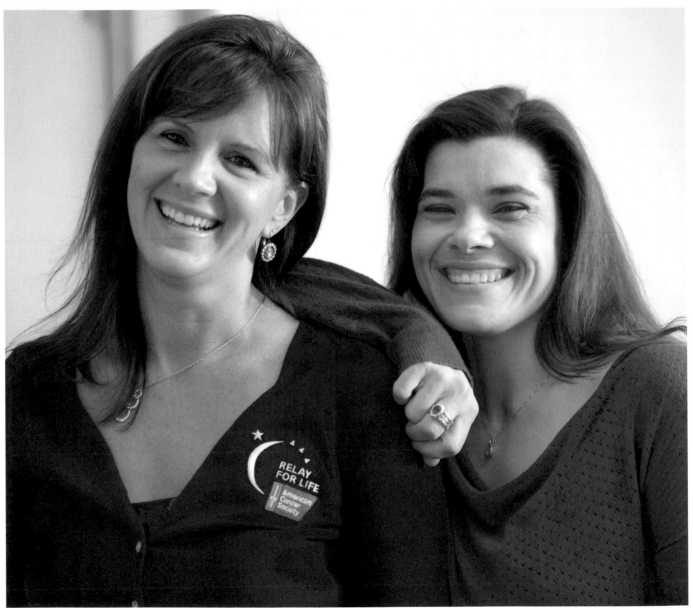

Nicole Messier, RN, BSN, with Amy Deavitt [right]

care of me. There was a lot we did not know. But what we did know was that I was a 32-year-old woman with invasive ductal breast cancer, that we had the best of the best our hospital had to offer and that Nicole was leading the charge.

The day after my mastectomy, Nicole was by my bedside, assuring me that the drain tubes I was complaining so heavily about would be much easier to handle with the shirts she had brought me that had special pockets to place the bulbs in. She also had instructions for me on how to shower and care for them. She had the skill to make everything seem a little easier. I became quite certain that with Nicole by our side, cancer did not stand a chance.

The days turned into weeks, and it was time to have the tubes out. Unfortunately, because my husband had been missing so much work, he was not able to be with me for this procedure. I had shared that with Nicole when she called that morning to congratulate me on getting the tubes out. It did not surprise me to see the door open and Nicole walk in just as the first tube was to be pulled.

TEACHING MOMENT:

I knew firsthand how important it was to see our nurses outside of the medical facilities they treat us in and how important it was to see them at our local relay. Without a second thought, Nicole joined forces with me, and four years later, we are still growing our relay together.

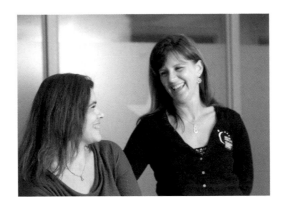

In 2006, I had a scare that landed me in the emergency room. I wanted so much to be treated like a "normal" patient, hoping they would not call in my team. It was the middle of the night; the team would not know. Just before eight the next morning, Nicole called to check in on me. How did she know? Well, they did contact my team, and Nicole and my doctor were trading emails early in the morning about me. It was then that I realized I was not going to walk alone in this fight.

I have never faced an appointment in my nine years that Nicole was not a part of in some way. Even though Nicole has since moved out of the Breast Cancer Clinic and was promoted to Clinical Program Coordinator of the Vermont Cancer Center, I know she is always only a phone call away.

By 2009, my life had changed. I had given up the business I had owned for 19 years and had begun working full time for the American Cancer Society. I had been volunteering for them since 2004, when I decided to fight back as a member of their Relay For Life. Nicole had even helped rally a group of doctors and nurses to attend a fundraiser I threw for our team. This time, I reached out to Nicole to help lead the mission education piece of my work. I knew firsthand how important it was to see our nurses outside of the medical facilities they treat us in and how important it was to see them at our local relay. Without a second thought, Nicole joined forces with me, and four years later, we are still growing our relay together.

With Nicole, I have had a medical adviser, nurse, caregiver and, most importantly, a lifelong friend. I am certain the care I have been given by Nicole has played a huge part in my ability to fight back with her as we work together toward a cure. ❧

2013 Extraordinary Healer Award for Oncology Nursing

Nominees

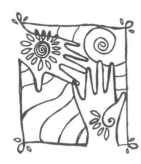

CURE congratulates each nurse who was nominated. You are all extraordinary healers.

Peggy Alton, RN, BSN, OCN / Duke University Medical Center

Lisa Armao, RN, FNP, ANP-C / Women's Cancer Care Associates

Jane Baggett, RN / VCU Massey Cancer Center

Pat Balzac, RN / Texas Oncology

Patti Barkley, RN, MS, ANP-C / MD Anderson Cancer Center

Christina Baumrucker Farrell, RN / Evanston Kellogg Cancer Center

Rob Beach, RN, OCN / Compass Oncology

Cynthia Bedell, RN, MSN, NP-C / Mary Crowley Cancer Research Centers

Juanita Bellinger, RN, OCN / Cancer Care Associates

Ellen Berg, RN, MSN, OCN / Rush-Copley Cancer Care Center

Dani Best, RN, BSN, OCN / Cancer Resource Center

Leslie Biggs, RN, OCN / Dorwart Cancer Care Center

Paige Brantley, RN, OCN / Tennessee Cancer Specialists

Jill Brown, RN, BSN, OCN / Wayne HealthCare

Pauline Buszkiewicz, RN / Massachusetts General Hospital

Kathy Byrne, RN / Boston Medical Center

Aryln Camacho, ARNP-BC / The Pancreatic & Biliary Center of South Florida

Andrea Cartmill, RN / Palo Verde Cancer Specialists

Carolina Caso, RN, BSN, CPON, OCN / Cedars-Sinai
Medical Center

Sally Celano, RN / Geisinger Community Medical Center

Deborah Czybora, RN / Boston Medical Center

Brenda Damiano, RN, MSN, CHPN / Hospice of New Jersey

Michael DeAngelo, RN, OCN / Thompson Oncology Center

Susan Deeney, RN, BSN, OCN / Burlington County
Hematology Oncology

Monica Del Rosso, RN, BSN, OCN / Orange Regional
Medical Center

Vanna Dest, MSN, APRN, BC, AOCN / Hospital of Saint
Raphael

Mary Dibley, RN, HP (ASCP) / James P. Wilmot Cancer
Center, University of Rochester Medical Center

Teri Dougherty, APN, NP / RUSH University Medical Center

Linda Dowling, RN, BSN, OCN / Illinois Cancer Specialists

Kyra Erwin, RN, BSN, CPHON / Seattle Children's Hospital

Pamela Fellenz, RN, ONC, CC, WCC / Mayo Clinic Health
System, Cancer Center

Lesley Ferguson, RN, OCN / Virginia Oncology Associates

Kitty Forbush, RN, BA / Pluta Cancer Center

Sherry Gangelhoff, RN, BSN / John T. Vucurevich Cancer
Care Institute

Margie Garity, RN / Boston Medical Center

Nancy Garner, RN / Boston Medical Center

Barbara Gregory, RN, OCN / Audrain Medical Center at SSM
Health Care

Peggy Guerrera, RN / Boston Medical Center

Patricia Hauck, RN, OCN / Chester County Hematology
Oncology Services, Chester County Hospital

Heather Hines, RN, OCN / University Hospitals Seidman
Cancer Center

Cynthia Hingle, RN, BSN, OCN / Slidell Memorial Hospital

Wanda Holsapple, RN / Premier Healthcare

Sara Joy, RN / MD Anderson Cancer Center

Laura Kennah, RN, OCN / Orlando VAMC

Michelle Knowles, APRN-BC / Tucker Gosnell Center
for Gastrointestinal Cancers, Massachusetts General
Hospital

Donna LaBarge, RN, BSN, OCN / The Ohio State University
Wexner Medical Center

Darlene Landi, RN / Hillman Cancer Center, UPMC

Aimee Lapierre-Hunt, RN / University of Colorado Cancer
Center

Connie Lass, RN, OCN / Josephine Ford Cancer Institute

Jo Ann Lawrence, RN, APN / The Valley Hospitals

Peggy Lawrie, RN / Medical Oncology & Hematology

Kim Nelles Lewis, RN, OCN, ONN / Coliseum Cancer Institute

James Linehan, RN, MS / Boston Medical Center

Joelle Link, RN, BSN / Penn Medicine, Hospital of the University of Pennsylvania

Diane Linn, RN / Texas Oncology

Karen Litwak, RN, ANP, APRN, AOCN / SUNY Upstate Regional Oncology Office

Sylvia Macco, RN / Stony Brook University Hospital

Jane Makson, RN / Boston Medical Center

Patricia Manea, RN, OCN, CRC / Cancer Care Center of South Texas

Suzanne McGettigan, CRNP / Abramson Cancer Center of the University of Pennsylvania

Mary Ann McKann, RN / Saratoga Hospital

Patricia McKinney, RN, BSN, OCN / Novant Health Breast Center, Huntersville

Maureen Meisel, RN / Boston Medical Center

Nicole Messier, RN, BSN / Vermont Cancer Center

Debbie Miller, RN, OCN / Mary Bird Perkins Cancer Center at Tammany Parish Hospital

Victoria Miller, RN, BSN, OCN / Kaiser Permanente

Beverly Moser, RN, BSN, OCN / Compass Oncology, Rose Quarter Office

Dawn Motes, CMSRN / Crescent City Physicians

Maria Pilar Nagy, RN, ACLS, PALS / Sacred Heart Medical Oncology Group

Colleen O'Brien, RN, CBCN, CBPN-IC / Winthrop-University Hospital Breast Health Center

Melinda Perritt, BSN, OCN / Zimmer Cancer Center, New Hanover Regional Medical Center

Robin Petro, RN, BSN / Comprehensive Cancer Center at Wake Forest Baptist Medical Center

Chris Piper, RN, OCN / John T. Vucurevich Cancer Care Institute

Victoria Poillucci, RN, MSN, ACNP-BC, ANP / Preston Robert Tisch Brain Tumor Center, Duke

Carlene Porter, APN, CNP / Cadence Physician Group

Debbi Pothmann, LPN / Office of Michael Greenhawt, MD, Memorial Cancer Institute

Gail Probst, RN, MS, ANP, AOCN, NE-BC / Huntington Hospital

Teresa Pugliese, RN / Boston Medical Center

Ann Puglisi, RN, BSN, OCN / NorthShore University HealthSystem Kellogg Cancer Center

Lisa Quirk, RN, OCN / Yolanda G. Barco Oncology Institute, Meadville Medical Center

Dorothy Lippman Salovesh, ACHPN, SNP-BC, GNP-BC / St. Jude Medical Center

Cheryl Santosusso, RN, BSN / Jefferson Infusion Center at Kimmel Cancer Center, Thomas Jefferson University Hospital

Karen Sellner, RN / Mercy Oncology Hematology Center at Mercy Hospital

Patrick Silovich, RN, BSN / Masonic Cancer Center, University of Minnesota

Mary Kate Simon, RN / Boston Medical Center

Kathy Solari, RN / Kennedy Memorial Hospital

Rosebud Sserebe, RN / Massachusetts General Hospital

Sandra Steel, RN, BSN / Dartmouth-Hitchcock Norris Cotton Cancer Center

Robert H. Steele, RN, OCN / Compass Oncology

Joanne Stranieri, RN, OCN / Hospital of Central Connecticut

Carolyn Sweeney, RN, OCN / Banner MD Anderson Cancer Center

Diana Tam, RN, BSN, OCN / Memorial Sloan-Kettering Cancer Center

Jane Thompson, RN, BSN / Massachusetts General Hospital

Tahitia Timmons, MSN, RN-BC, OCN, VA-BC / Virtua Memorial

Nanette van der Sanden, RN, CMF / Commenci

Blanca Vargas, RN, BSN, OCN / Creticos Cancer Center, Advocate Illinois Masonic Medical Center

Angela Ward, NP / The Emory Clinic

Nancy Washburn, RN, MSN, ARNP, BC, ANP, AOCN, NP / University of Kansas Cancer Center

Cheri Wick, RN, BSN, OCN, CBCN / Providence St. Vincent Medical Center

Lori Willcoxon, RN, BSN, OCN / Missouri Cancer Associates

Monique Williams, RN, NP / Urology Cancer Clinic, University of Michigan

Vicki Wilson, RN / Arizona Oncology Associates

Jackie Woods, RN, OCN / Arizona Oncology Associates

Pamela Young, RN / Presence United Samaritans Regional Cancer Center